The Tactile Heart

Also by John M. Hull

Sense and Nonsense About God

Hellenistic Magic and the Synoptic Tradition

School Worship – An Obituary

Studies in Religion and Education

What Prevents Christian Adults from Learning?

The Act Unpacked: The Meaning of the 1988 Education Reform Act for Religious Education

Touching the Rock: An Experience of Blindness

God-Talk with Young Children

Mishmash: Religious Education in Multi-Cultural Britain, A Study in Metaphor

On Sight and Insight: A Journey into the World of Blindness

Utopian Whispers: Moral, Religious and Spiritual Values in Schools

In the Beginning There Was Darkness: A Blind Person's Conversations with the Bible

Mission-Shaped Church: A Theological Response

The Tactile Heart

Blindness and Faith

John M. Hull

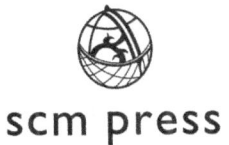

scm press

© John M. Hull 2013

Published in 2013 by SCM Press
Editorial office
3rd Floor
Invicta House
108–114 Golden Lane,
London
EC1Y 0TG

SCM Press is an imprint of Hymns Ancient & Modern Ltd
(a registered charity)
13A Hellesdon Park Road
Norwich NR6 5DR, UK

www.scmpress.co.uk

All rights reserved. No part of this publication may be reproduced,
stored in a retrieval system, or transmitted,
in any form or by any means, electronic, mechanical,
photocopying or otherwise, without the prior permission of
the publisher, SCM Press.

Scripture quotations are from the New Revised Standard Version of
the Bible, copyright 1989 by the Division of Christian Education of the
National Council of Churches of Christ in the USA. Used by permission.

The Author has asserted his right under the Copyright, Designs and
Patents Act, 1988, to be identified as the Author of this Work

British Library Cataloguing in Publication data

A catalogue record for this book is available
from the British Library

978 0 334 04933 3

Typeset by Regent Typesetting, London
Printed and bound by
CPI Group (UK) Ltd, Croydon

Contents

Preface vii

1. The Tactile Heart — 1
2. Milton, *Paradise Lost* and Blindness — 4
3. The Material Spirituality of Blindness and Money — 9
4. Open Letter from a Blind Disciple to a Sighted Saviour: Text and Discussion — 13
5. Blindness and the Face of God: Toward a Theology of Disability — 42
6. A Spirituality of Disability: The Christian Heritage as Both Problem and Potential — 59
7. Is Blindness a World? From Theology of Impairment to Theology of Disability — 77
8. The Broken Body in a Broken World: A Contribution to a Christian Doctrine of the Person from a Disabled Point of View — 90
9. 'Sight to the Inly Blind'? Attitudes to Blindness in the Hymnbooks — 112
10. 'Lord, I was Deaf': Images of Disability in the Hymnbooks — 124
11. Teaching as a Trans-world Activity — 143

Acknowledgements of Previous Publication 152

For Marilyn

I hate all sighted things but for your sake I love them.
It was because of you that I embraced blindness;
You gave me strength to turn from the world of nostalgic
  images
And face the dark future where you are.
I hate the darkness that hides me from you
And I hate the light which hides you from me.

I love both worlds, yours and mine
And so across the worlds, I love you.

Preface

I became a registered blind person in August 1980. It did not occur to me that there was anything particularly interesting or remarkable about blindness; it was all perfectly straightforward although admittedly most inconvenient: blindness is when your eyes don't work and you need to find other ways of doing things. Three years later my attitude changed. The last traces of light sensation had faded, and the lingering hope of some slight improvement had been crushed. I was now disorientated in the world, not only by what blindness was doing to me but by the nature of blindness itself. I did not set out to write about blindness. My first book on this subject, *Touching the Rock: An Experience of Blindness* (1990), was based upon a series of tape recordings made over a number of years in order to enable me to monitor and meditate upon the changes that were taking place. These original recordings from the mid-1980s have now been retrieved by Fee Fie Foe Films, who are using them as the basis of a film about blindness which will be released in 2014 or 2015 under the title *Into Darkness*. An enlarged second edition of *Touching the Rock* was published in 1997 under the title *On Sight and Insight*. The original *Touching the Rock* was republished as an SPCK Classic in May 2013.

Although the experience of blindness changed the way I thought of God, it was not a challenge to my faith, so much as to my imagination. The imagery of light was replaced by the more intimate meanings of darkness. When I read the Bible as a blind person, however, it was a different matter. *In the Beginning There was Darkness: A Blind Person's Conversations with the Bible* (2001) describes how I came to realize that the

Bible was mostly written by sighted people. The disturbing fact that the Gospels portrayed Jesus as a sighted person sharing the usual first-century attitudes towards blindness came as a shock. My earlier reflections had been of a personal nature but now the foundations were laid for a more thoughtful theology of blindness. This took the shape of a number of reflections upon Christian faith including some analysis of the phenomenology of the blind condition and its significance for social and ethical living.

This present book, *The Tactile Heart: Studies in Blindness and Faith*, is a collection of these studies, most of which have been published as book chapters and periodical articles although a couple are appearing here for the first time. These meditations on sightlessness, now spread over 30 years, have moved from the autobiographical, in which I tried to understand myself, to the biblical, in which I tried to understand Scripture, and now to a more mature but still fragmentary series of reflections upon the deeper meaning of blindness for the religious life.

I am grateful to the RNIB who in 2012 presented me with a lifetime achievement award for contributions to the literature of blindness, and to The Allan & Nesta Ferguson Charitable Trust and the Westhill Endowment Trust, whose generous support has made this work possible. I am also grateful to Natalie Watson of the SCM Press for her careful work in preparing the text.

These writings on blindness have been the subject of music, drama, poetry and works of art, which have given a wider scope to my intentions of bridging the blind and sighted worlds and of interpreting one to the other. The most profound and redemptive experience of these two worlds has been my relationship with Marilyn, to whom this book is dedicated.

John M. Hull
The Queen's Foundation for
Ecumenical Theological Education
Birmingham

I

The Tactile Heart

The beauties of touch are, I suppose, largely hidden from many sighted people. For those who go blind in adult life, the loss of beauty must be one of the most perplexing problems. Those in the blind state who do not wish to remain as sighted people who cannot see, but to become authentic blind people, will find that discovering the beauty of touch is one of their most important tasks.

In my own experience – perhaps I am not alone in this – one passes through three stages in the learning of tactile beauty. First, there is the stage when, with our hands, we learn again to do. There is the second stage when, with our hands, we learn to know. Finally, there is that stage when, with our hands, we learn to appreciate beauty.

The first stage, the doing stage, is in itself sufficiently perplexing. So accustomed are sighted people to think of the eye and the hand as being interlocked that the separation of the eye from the hand, which is the condition of blindness, causes considerable puzzlement. It takes time for both blind and sighted to realize that you don't have to see to do up your shoelaces, to brush your teeth or put on your tie, although I must admit that it helps a little to know what tie you are putting on. It takes time to realize that, as a blind person trying to unlock a door, you have to remember what it was like coming home late at night drunk. You need one hand to locate the keyhole and the other hand to shove the key in. This is an example of blind doing.

When one has rediscovered blind doing through the hand, the next stage is more difficult. To move on to blind knowing is so much more complex. Of course, sighted people do use their hands for knowing. One licks one's finger and sticks it up in a breeze. One touches something to discover whether or not it is hot, and one says 'ouch'. These experiences are relatively isolated for the sighted. In the case of the blind, we see with our fingers more regularly. For us, tactile knowing is our standard form of knowledge.

It is surprising, for those who lose sight, how difficult this is, although for those blind from birth it is, of course, their natural form of knowledge. I well remember, as a recently blinded person, learning again to play chess with my children. How difficult I found it to remember that in the case of the blind one not only moves the pieces with one's fingers; one knows the whole structure of the board with one's fingers. One must not try to hold in one's imagination a picture of the board with its black and white pieces, but one must learn to play the game with one's hands. One must let the hands solve that intricate puzzle of tiny relationships which is typical of tactile knowing.

In the last month, I have started to learn to play the piano. As I explore my major musical achievement so far, which is the key of C in contrary motion, I try to repress that image of the black and white notes of the keyboard which keeps coming before my mind. My hands are beyond light and darkness. To me it is nothing that there are black and white keys. My fingers have to learn that the keys are grouped in bunches spread out in rows across a space; some stick up and some are flat. They are arranged into these little groups of twos and threes. This is what my hands know and this is the way my mind has to work to play the piano. I must, in other words, have a tactile brain which will match my tactile form of knowing.

When we arrive at the third stage, the stage of discovering tactile beauty, we reach realms that are yet more subtle. Here, I think, there is not such a difference between those born blind and those who have lost some sight or all sight later in life. Just as sighted people need continual education in how to appreciate visual beauty, so blind people of all kinds need education in order to appreciate tactile beauty. It is foolish for blind people to sit around bemoaning the loss of the moon and the mountain. For us, beauty is more intimate, more concrete, more immediate, more particular. Gradually the blind rediscover the beauty of ordinary things. In the world of blind beauty we rediscover the loveliness of cups and saucers, of milk bottles and teaspoons, of rocks and bricks, of the bark of trees and the feel of human hair.

One of the remarkable things about tactile beauty is the element of surprise. I admit that not all tactile surprise is particularly beautiful, and I have frequently been surprised by a very tactile encounter with a lamp-post or the edge of a door. Nevertheless, one of the treasures of blindness is the great capacity to be surprised by joy. A dozen times a day we blind people find ourselves holding something in our hands, whether it is a cat or a cushion, and saying, 'Oh, so that's what it's like.' That capacity for immediate surprise is one of the delights of the tactile beauty which is only accessible to the blind.

I have spoken of the tactile brain. Now I would like to move on to the tactile heart, because, although we know with our brains, we feel with our hearts. How interesting that we should feel both with our fingers and with our hearts! It may be that in the case of the totally blind the intimate link between the eye and the finger is broken, but the other equally intimate connection between the finger and the heart may be restored.

Let us think how the tactile heart is used in religious imagination to express our response to God. In tactile doing, knowing and appreciating beauty, we find metaphors of our human condition before God. Do you remember how the Lord God made us human beings in the first place? Did God not kneel down in the dust of the earth and use fingers to mould us? Did God not hold us, warm against God's own body, and breathe into us the breath of life? So we became living men and women. We are close to the heart of this tactile God.

Do we not remember those stories about Jesus Christ? His contemporaries were amazed because he touched people. He touched the untouchable, the unlovely, the poor and the sick. He laid his hands upon little children. Moreover, he made himself available to be touched, for to touch is to be touched. So it was that Thomas was invited to touch his hands and his side, and when the first Christians looked back and described the experience they had had of God in Christ, they spoke of that which they had touched with their hands (1 John 1.1).

2

Milton, *Paradise Lost* and Blindness

Blind and sighted people experience the world in such different ways that it is quite difficult for one to really understand the other. *Paradise Lost* was written by a blind person but its readers are usually sighted people. For most of these, the fact that John Milton was blind would be no more than a passing thought, mixed, perhaps, with some curiosity about how he managed to do it, and the compassion that is characteristic of the attitude of sighted people towards blind friends, but no more. It would not occur to many sighted people that blindness itself might be a significant clue to understanding the poem.

To be more precise, the poem is not so much about blindness as about the experience of losing sight in adult life. This is described first in all the horror and despair of the initial impact, and then with a kind of calm and accepting sadness. The first phase is depicted as the loss of heaven and the fall into the abyss, and the second phase is represented by the loss of the garden of paradise and the mixture of resignation and hope with which a new kind of world is faced.

As Satan, the blind Milton falls from the world of light into a place where

> A dungeon horrible, on all sides round
> As one great furnace flamed, yet from those flames
> No light, but rather darkness visible ...[1]

---

[1] John Milton, *Paradise Lost*, introduced by Philip Pullman, Oxford: Oxford University Press, 2005, Bk I: ll. 61–63.

When you lose your sight, it is as if the world has closed in upon you; you are trapped inside your body feeling the claustrophobia of a 'prison ordained / In utter darkness', 'far removed from God and light of heaven', made worse by the painful memory of the past: 'O how unlike the place from which they fell!'[2]

The question is then whether to bow your head and sink into passivity, or whether to find

> courage never to submit or yield:
> And what is else not to be overcome?[3]

It has been said that sighted people live in the world, but blind people live in their minds, 'for the mind and spirit remains / Invincible, and vigour soon returns'[4] and one learns that

> The mind is its own place, and in itself
> Can make a heaven of hell, a hell of heaven.[5]

The result is the building of the great assembly hall, ironically named Pandemonium; the title is conferred from the point of view of the outsiders, for although it is created in 'The prison of his tyranny',[6] it does restore order and a sense of place. This is surely none other than the great poem itself in all its majestic architecture and complex structure. I understand a little of this, because when I lost my sight and had to speak in public without notes, I had to become very systematic in my mind, otherwise I lost the thread, and so did my hearers!

The second account of loss is also described as a fall. It represents a later stage in the grieving process which accompanies the onset of blindness. No less dramatic than the fall into hell, it is marked by elements of acceptance and even penitence. But why penitence? True, one is not to be blamed for one's blindness, and yet many a man must have felt that in his inability to

---

2 Bk I: ll. 71–75.
3 Bk I: ll. 108–109.
4 Bk I: ll. 139–140.
5 Bk I: ll. 254–255.
6 Bk II: l. 59.

defend his wife and to control his children he has descended into 'this dark opprobrius den of shame'.⁷ And why guilt? Irrational though it is, many a blinded person must have asked, 'What did I do to deserve this?' It is emotions such as these that lie behind the whole conception of blindness as an explusion, a fall and a punishment.

In the second phase of the experience of losing sight, the poet contemplates the loss of the everyday things of life:

> ... but not to me returns
> Day, or the sweet approach of even or morn,
> Or sight of vernal bloom, or summer's rose,
> Or flocks, or herds, or human face divine;
> But cloud instead, and ever-during dark
> Surrounds me, from the cheerful ways of men
> Cut off, and for the world of knowledge fair
> Presented with a universal blank ...⁸

Sight is now a garden of innocence, beauty and sexual freedom. The blind poet fantasizes about the loss of the exuberant motion and different shapes of the animal world, and the loss of the visual delight of flowers, and the sunsets he recalls

> Arraying with reflected purple and gold
> The clouds that on his western throne attend ...⁹

Most of all he mourns the loss of the beauty of the female figure, and the centrepiece of his wistful memory is the freedom and innocence of making love in the open air. How wonderful it would be to be with the most lovely woman in the world – indeed, the only woman in the world – and to possess her in the security of knowing that there were no prying eyes, but for the angelic guards!

But now all that is gone for ever and there is no point in bold defiance, for

---

7 Bk II: l. 58.
8 Bk III: ll. 41–47.
9 Bk IV: ll. 596–597.

> ... prayer against his absolute decree
> No more avails than breath against the wind
> ... Therefore to his great bidding I submit.[10]

But what about the face of God?

> This most afflicts me, that departing hence,
> As from his face I shall be hid, deprived
> His blessed countenance ...[11]

Where is God for blind people? So much of the imagery with which the divine is depicted is visual!
But there is comfort.

> ... surmise not then
> His presence to these narrow bounds confined ...[12]

There may be a kind of restoration, and Adam becomes, like his master Milton, a blind seer.

> ... but to nobler sights
> Michael from Adam's eyes the film removed
> Which that false fruit that promised clearer sight
> Had bred; then purged with euphrasy and rue
> The visual nerve, for he had much to see;
> And from the well of life three drops instilled.
> So deep the power of these ingredients pierced,
> Even to the inmost seat of mental sight ...[13]

Thus the angel of prophecy is hailed as 'True opener of my eyes!'[14]
The lesson to be learned is that

---

10 Bk XI: ll. 311–314.
11 Bk XI: ll. 315–317.
12 Bk XI: ll. 340–341.
13 Bk XI: ll. 411–418.
14 Bk XI: l. 598.

> ... suffering for truth's sake
> Is fortitude to highest victory,
> And to the faithful death the gate of life.[15]

Michael, the archangel, assures Adam that he will find 'A Paradise within'.[16]

There is a world before him, less predictable and more dangerous than the previous one, in which he and his partner are more vulnerable and more alone. Nevertheless, hand in hand they face the future with courage and hope.

What are we today to make of this double experience of blindness? *Paradise Lost* describes three worlds, one of majesty and power, one of desperation and utter loss, and the third a world of quiet acceptance, where the inner vision of the mind can still converse with angels. The elements of guilt, self-accusation and social rejection are still experienced by many blind people today although it is possible that our more inclusive and multi-cultural society is beginning to realize that there are many human worlds. Blindness is, no doubt, a smaller world, and those entering it may still experience it as a fall, but the little blind world is not without its own integrity and autonomy. And within that world much may still be achieved.

---

15 Bk XII: ll. 569–571.
16 Bk XII: l. 587.

3

The Material Spirituality of Blindness and Money

We have the spirituality which is in the interests of the people with whom we stand in solidarity. The wealthy and powerful are embedded within a spirituality that consciously or not contributes to maintain their interests in the world. This is because our spirituality, made up as it is of our self-ideals, our hopes and dreams, our interpretation of our place in the world and our relationship with others, together with our perception of the transcendent meaning of our lives, necessarily reflects our position in society.

For many years, I did not know this. In my childhood and youth, I was enclosed within a spirituality that concentrated upon the personal presence of Jesus as I experienced him in the evangelical Christian faith. It did not occur to me that this spirituality had its own history. I just thought it was true.

Due partly to theological study and partly to a wider experience of life, I realized that the spirituality of my childhood was itself an artefact of my upbringing, an expression of a certain moment in the history of Christian faith, realized by me at a certain period of my own life. I began to be spiritually critical of my spirituality. Gradually, I adopted the spirituality appropriate to a theological lecturer, a mixture of critical commitment, enquiry, and an interest in the personal growth of my students. I had a spirituality of meaning, in the sense that my main understanding of Christian faith was that it offered meaning to our lives.

Then I went blind. I realized that my consciousness as a sighted person had not been absolute, but was limited and had given me a certain point of view upon the world. I realized that the Bible had been written by sighted people and for sighted people, and that I as sighted had been embedded within this obvious spirituality, to emerge from which had not even occurred to me.

During those years, I had become interested in false consciousness and self-deception as elements in spirituality. I was increasingly successful in my career, receiving several promotions and rising to senior management in the institution where I worked. At the same time, however, I realized that false consciousness was creeping up my life like a rising tide. It became easier to see life from the top of the pile and more difficult to imagine it from underneath. It was blindness that saved me from completely succumbing to this fatal falseness. Facing every day a dozen frustrations and little humiliations, continually aware of my dependence upon others, alienated at the same time from an easy rapport with other people, I became increasingly conscious of the way that marginalized and disabled people experience the world.

Then it dawned upon me that the greatest spiritual force in the world today is money. Nothing affects our imagining of the good life and the way we mould our ambitions so as to attain it as does money. I realized that as a blind person I had to have money, and I understood how terrible was the plight of blind men with families.

Previously I had thought that spirituality comes down from above, from God, or from a supposed spiritual world, from another world which I had conceived of as being transcendent over the actual world in which I and other people lived. Now I began, slowly, to realize that spirituality comes up from below. I understood now that blindness was not only something that happened to your eyes or to your brain or to your body, but was a world-creating condition. Sight is also a world-creating condition, but sighted people do not usually realize this. They think the world is just like that. Now I understood that I was being compelled to live in a new world, a world created by blindness, where time and people and the difference between the conscious and the unconscious life were all reconstituted. This world was created by my blindness in the sense that it was projected from my blind body.

Spirituality, by which I mean the way we constitute our human relationships, our sense of time and space, our realization of selfhood and so on, comes up from below. These realities are created for us by the relationship between our bodies and the world, by the relationship between our lives and our bodies in the material context of life. Formerly a heavenly spiritualist, I now became a spiritual materialist. Then I understood that what was true of blindness and its power to create a spiritual world was also true of money, which as the objective realization of the human will and the concrete expression of relationships generates its own real world. Money creates its own culture. In so far as this money-culture influences self-esteem, our scale of values, our motivations, our ideas of God, it can be said to produce a kind of spirituality. In so far as money has become the main instrument of exploitation and oppression, the spirituality of the money-culture that we have today must be denounced as a false spirituality, and a principal task of the Christian faith is to unmask the deceptions and especially the self-deceptions with which the money-culture conceals itself.

And so, gradually I felt my way towards a spirituality of justice. I came to see that the search for justice and the struggle against the forces of money which prevent universal justice is the way God is known. This is the transcendent element in our living, the particularities of concrete justice in solidarity with others.

Implementing this in my life presents me with a continual series of new falsehoods and further layers of self-deception. I seek to remove these by a series of tiny steps, each one of which restores my sense of spiritual balance. I know that these steps are only a beginning but, as a blind person and someone seeking, however feebly, to live an ethical life, I have learned a spirituality of taking one step at a time. This itself can be an excuse for not taking two steps.

However, beneath this I believe that I am somehow sustained by a love and a grace which is both smaller than me and greater than me.

It is smaller than me because it pays attention to every detail. The life of a blind person is crowded with details so small that sighted people seldom notice them. It is greater than me because it is the environment in which I live. The life of a sighted person is set within realities, like stars, hills and cities, which are almost too large to be realized. When I discovered the marble altar in Iona Abbey, in the island of Iona off the coast of Scotland, in the middle of the night, I found that there were jagged scratches on either side of which the expanse of polished stone stretched smooth as silk further than I could reach. This surface was made by people, but in the excoriations there was something older and deeper, a rock not cut by hands. Which was the small and which the great? The scratches were small and the surface was great, yet the altar was small and the rock was great.

4

Open Letter from a Blind Disciple to a Sighted Saviour

Text and Discussion

Introduction

When I wrote about the miracles of Jesus, nearly 40 years ago, I approached the problem from a critical historical point of view.[1] I was primarily interested in the world out of which the text came. I tried to set my work within the context of similar critical scholarship and that is why there were lots of footnotes. It did not occur to me to ask how blind or deaf people might react to my discussion of the healing miracles. In that respect, things have not changed much. While writing my 'Open Letter to Jesus' (see below), I studied about a dozen articles written in the tradition of critical historical exegesis.[2] I noticed as a blind person what I had not seen when I was sighted, that the people, presumably mostly sighted, who write articles about the symbolism of blindness in the Gospels never seem to reflect upon the implications of this for blind people.

In my 'Open Letter to Jesus', I deliberately adopted a different approach. I concentrated not upon the world out of which the texts came, but upon the world which the texts tended to create, the horizon towards which they seemed to point.[3] I tried

---

[1] John M. Hull, *Hellenistic Magic and the Synoptic Tradition*, London: SCM Press, 1974.

[2] For example, E. S. Johnson, 'Mark X: 46–52 Blind Bartimaeus', *Catholic Biblical Quarterly* 40 (1978), pp. 191–204.

[3] Paul Ricœur, *Interpretation Theory: Discourse and the Surplus of Meaning*, Fort Worth: Texas Christian University, 1976, pp. 36f.

to bracket out my previous familiarity with the Bible, to forget the meaning which many of those passages had had for me in my former sighted life and to allow the biblical speech (I did it all on tape) to fall into my consciousness like rain upon the dry ground.[4]

It did not seem to make any difference to my response to the text, as I heard it, whether the words of Jesus about the Pharisees being 'blind fools' are due to Matthew's editorial construction rather than being close to something Jesus may actually have said. For the same reason, I did not always study the Gospel parallels and variants in cases where a saying or story appears more than once. I simply responded to what my tape-recorder was reading to me. However, in describing how a *particular* blind person reacts to the Bible, I believe that I have shown something about the Bible *in general* and not only something about myself.

My method of interpretation is typical of post-modern responses to the meaning of the Bible.[5] Now that we have learned from Asian, African and South American biblical interpretation, to say nothing of feminist and black readings, we realize that the tradition of European biblical scholarship has European characteristics.[6] Just as we have theology that represents the interests of the people with whom we stand in solidarity, so we have the Bible that sustains that solidarity. All knowledge is within the circle of human interest, and there is no unmotivated truth.[7] Nevertheless, when we understand that the knowledge and the truth about the Bible is driven by the socio-historical position of the commentators, and that 'the meaning of the Bible' is necessarily a cultural artefact, we are invited to put that meaning against the meanings of the Bible from other socio-cultural positions. The sighted truth about the Bible may be true and yet

---

4 The result is a hermeneutic similar to that which Kwok Pui-Lan describes as 'the Bible as a talking book'. Kwok Pui-Lan, *Discovering the Bible in the Non-Biblical World*, Maryknoll: Orbis, 1995, pp. 40–3.

5 Walter Brueggemann, *The Bible and Post-Modern Imagination: Texts Under Negotiation*, London: SCM Press, 1993.

6 R. S. Sugirtharajah, *Voices From the Margin: Interpreting the Bible in the Third World*, London: SPCK, 1995.

7 Jürgen Habermas, *Knowledge and Human Interests*, London: Heinemann Educational, 1978.

not all the truth. In so far as it is not the complete truth, we are misled if we absolutize it.

This, then, is an attempt to relativize or pluralize the Bible. Without denying the truth that the Bible is mainly a book for sighted people, I want to relativize that truth by making it obvious, and by stating the obvious to relativize it.[8] The truth that the Bible is a book for sighted people is related to the truth that the Bible is also a book for blind people. If the Bible is relatively a book for sighted people, then the Bible is also relatively a book for men, for hearing people, for white people and for wealthy people, and so on. Is there no end to this process of relativization? Is there, after all, no absolute truth in the Bible?

If there is an absolute truth, it is not to be found through a process of artificial and often unconscious absolutizing, but through a proliferation of many meanings until everyone's meanings are gathered in. This is the way that the Bible becomes truly ecumenical, truly catholic. We do not know how many more perspectives there might be. We do not know how many new groups and new cultures will hold up the diamond of God's word and give it a new twist, so that new patterns and colours flash forth from it; but if the Bible is to be a book for all people, this process cannot be arrested. It is necessary that all those who are spoken to by the Bible should have an opportunity to reply, and thus the conversation that is within the Bible can enter into conversation with us today, and, through offering a voice and a hearing to everyone, we can create a community of genuine free speech.[9]

In what sense can we say any longer that the Bible is the word of God? When I hear Jesus saying that the blind cannot lead the blind because they will both fall into a ditch, is that the word of God to me? When the Bible as a whole and the Gospels in particular, every one of them, tell me that as a blind person I represent disobedience, unbelief, ignorance and sin, am I to take that as God's word to me? This is not a word of acceptance, of

---

8 Michel Pêcheux, *Language, Semantics and Ideology: Stating the Obvious*, London: Macmillan, 1982.

9 Jürgen Habermas, *The Theory of Communicative Action*, 2 volumes, Boston, MA: Beacon Press, 1984, 1987.

forgiveness and of liberation, but a word of rejection, of oppression. In order to translate this into the word of God, we need to take out the disparaging metaphors. The truth to which faith witnesses is that our ignorance, sin and disobedience prevent us from responding to the love of God made known in Jesus Christ. It is not necessary that this witness of faith should be cast into the form of the metaphor of blindness. This is surely a case where the metaphor kills but the spirit gives life.

There are Christians who say that they believe the Bible to be literally true. Such Christians may find it difficult to recognize the metaphor of blindness and may be obliged by the nature of their faith in the authority of the Bible to adopt a condemnatory attitude towards blind people. This is the stark choice facing the biblical literalist: if you accept the Bible literally you will be more likely to accept uncritically the negative image of blindness in our culture.

We may make a similar comment about the speech of Jesus himself. When Jesus is reported to have said that the blind cannot lead the blind because they will both fall into a ditch, he means that people without understanding cannot become teachers of others without understanding because in that case neither will finish up with any understanding. It is not necessary to the truth spoken by Jesus that the metaphor of blindness should be used. When Jesus warned that the salt would be no good if it lost its saltiness, he was not speaking only about salt but about the presence of the teaching of the Kingdom of God in human lives. Nevertheless, we have to face the fact that to Jesus is attributed the use of a disparaging metaphor, a belittling and demeaning description which has oppressed and marginalized blind people down the centuries, because most Christians, even when they saw the truth beneath the metaphor, did not explicitly reject the metaphor, and therefore the text continued to collaborate in the building up of the cultural artefact in which blindness is belittled. As a free person in Christ and as a Christian blind person I lay this solemn charge against the Bible and against its sighted Christian interpreters.

Jesus used the metaphor, or the New Testament tradition attributed the use of the metaphor to Jesus, because the metaphor not only illustrated the truth but was believed to contain the truth. It was believed that blind people tended to be foolish, ignorant and inconsistent. If Jesus had said, 'The blind cannot lead the blind because they will both fall into a ditch but they don't really, I'm only trying to make a point,' the whole impact of the saying would have been lost. It would be like saying that the salt would be no good if it lost its saltiness – but it would be really.

The traditional authority of the Bible is now challenged on ethical as well as scientific grounds. The authority of the Bible must be evaluated in different ways. The Bible is a conversation into which we, who hear it, are drawn. It is a conversation in which we hear many voices – the rich and powerful, the poor and the oppressed. The Bible is the word of God because in it the voices of the poor and the oppressed have never been silenced.[10] We hear the voices of sighted people and, now and again, in a softer tone, the voices of blind people. The Bible is the word of God because, when we understand it in terms of its own variety and not through the perspective of our own enclosed biological and social conditions, it speaks to us not only as sighted people and blind people but as people. The biblical question is what we do with our sight, and what we do with our blindness.

I have chosen the genre of the open letter because it is an effective medium through which I can illustrate clearly and in an autobiographical way how I, as a blind person, react to the theme of blindness in the Bible and, in so doing, ensure that the Bible reveals its riches to everyone and not just to the sighted.

Open Letter to Jesus

Dear Jesus

According to the Gospel of Matthew, you used the expression 'blind' as a term of abuse. When you were attacking certain groups of people you described them as 'blind guides' (Matt.

---

10 George Thompson, *The First Philosophers*, London: Lawrence and Wishart, 1955, pp. 333ff. Ernst Bloch, *Atheism in Christianity: The Religion of the Exodus and the Kingdom*, New York: Herder & Herder, 1972.

23.16), 'blind fools' (v. 17), and 'you blind Pharisee' (v. 26). You have given your authority to those down the ages who have disparaged others through references to visual loss. Whenever a Member of Parliament criticizes a government minister by saying that he or she shows a blind disregard for the welfare of the people of this country, whenever a sports journalist describes a cricketer as having struck out blindly with the bat, or an academic recommends blind marking, the impression is reinforced that blind people are stubborn, callous, lacking in self-control or just plain ignorant. It would have been so easy for you to have called them 'careless guides', 'stupid fools', or 'stubborn Pharisees'. If you had spoken in that way, then the disparaging image of blindness, which has caused blind people so much pain, would not have received your permission and encouragement.

When I discuss these sayings with your sighted priests and other well-meaning friends, they defend you by pointing out that your use of the expression 'blind' is only metaphorical, but I cannot understand how this is supposed to help. In general, the Gospels show you as being sensitive and attentive to blind people (Mark 8.22–26; 10.46–52), so I cannot imagine that, if the guides, lawyers and Pharisees had been literally blind, you would have been so tactless as to refer to their blindness when criticizing them. Indeed, the problem is created precisely by the metaphorical use of blindness to suggest ignorance, stupidity and insensitivity.

Another point which your sighted friends make is that the disparaging use of blindness is confined to Matthew. The comparable passages in Mark and Luke do not use the expression 'blind' (Mark 12.38–40; Luke 20.45–47). We can conclude, the argument goes, that these references are to be attributed to Matthew himself or to the tradition upon which he was drawing, and not to you personally.

Well, perhaps that helps a little, but on the other hand I am not at all sure that there are many sayings in any of the Gospels which represent your actual words, and in any case, the offending words are part of Scripture, part of the picture which the first evangelist offers of you. When we hear these words read in church, we respond by saying 'Praise to Christ our Lord'. So whether you actually used the words or not, or said something like them in Aramaic, if not in Greek, you are nevertheless implicated in these texts.

The problem goes deeper than the mere disparaging use of the word 'blind'. When you referred to the blind guides, you illustrated the point by saying that they strained out a gnat and swallowed a camel (Matt. 23.24). In other words, the guides are fussy about details but overlook important things. This illustration becomes more significant in the context of the eating habits of blind people. If you sat with me at a table, Jesus, would you notice that, although I managed to eat the last pea on the plate, I completely ignored my glass of wine, because no one had told me it was there? Would you notice how I bit into the little pat of butter wrapped up in paper, which had been placed on top of my bread roll, and failed to notice the bowl of sauce into which I was supposed to dip my carrot sticks? You will remember, Lord, how in the early days of my blindness, when I was desperately trying to appear to be independent, I went along the buffet table indiscriminately, finishing up with sherry trifle on my roast vegetables.

The same sighted person's observation of blind people's behaviour is evident in the remark about first cleaning the inside of the cup and then the outside. The blind Pharisee is accused of washing the outside of the cups but ignoring the inside (Matt. 23.25). If you came to my office and shared a coffee with me, Jesus, would you be watching nervously to see whether the coffee cups were nice and clean? After all, the only way a blind person can know this is by feeling the inside of the cup, but most people do not like to drink from a cup the inside of which has been felt by someone else's sticky fingers. A blind person has to wash the cup every time to make sure it is clean, or keep the clean cups in a different place, or turn them upside down when they are washed. These techniques illustrate the difficulty of cleaning the inside as well as the outside. The fact that these observations are coupled with the accusation of blindness indicates that the word 'blind' is not used casually or accidentally, but arises from detailed observation of the behaviour of blind people. Oh dear, that makes it worse.

The truth is that in the days of your earthly ministry, my Lord, you were a sighted person. You naturally grew into the view of blind people that your sighted society conveyed to you. For example, Matthew says that you said of the Pharisees, 'Let them alone; they are blind guides of the blind. And if one blind person guides another, both will fall into a pit' (Matt. 15.14). I wonder that you should have said this, Lord, because your own experience of blind people leading each other suggested otherwise. In his ninth chapter, your evangelist Matthew describes how two blind men followed you and caught up with you when you entered into a house (Matt. 9.27–31). They must have followed the noisy crowd as it passed by and managed to catch up with you when you finally went into a house. They did not fall into a pit or a ditch. Moreover, it is more difficult to attribute this saying to Matthew than to you yourself, since Luke also reports it. 'Can a blind person lead a blind person? Will they not both fall into a pit?' (Luke 6.39). Luke introduces this comment as being a parable, but the parable would have derived its force from the fact that it was a genuine belief held among sighted people about the behaviour of blind people. You, my Lord, are described as participating in this general belief, but this says more about the assumptions and the prejudices of sighted people than about the actual behaviour of those who are blind. Blind people depend upon familiarity. A blind person who was familiar with a certain route would offer to lead a blind stranger along that way. I have myself led blind people many times and have in turn been led. We have never fallen into ditches, been run over on the road or fallen down stairs, although I admit to an occasional confrontation with a rose bush. It is when I am being led by a sighted person that I sometimes have bad experiences. As I am walking through a department store, the floor suddenly slides away from me and I almost lose my balance. 'Sorry,' my sighted friend says. 'I forgot to tell you that we are going down on the escalator.'

When I studied the New Testament as a sighted person, it did not occur to me that you, Jesus, were yourself sighted. We were in the same world, but it did not occur to me that being sighted was a world. I thought that things were just like that. When I became blind, then I realized that blindness is a world and that

FROM A BLIND DISCIPLE TO A SIGHTED SAVIOUR

the sighted condition also generates a distinctive experience and can be called a world. Now I find, Jesus, that I am in one world and you are in another.

This knowledge came to me for the first time when I read the Gospel of John as a blind person, but even then my understanding was limited. I encountered you in the Gospel of John with a sense of estrangement, because I realized as I read the Gospel in Braille, the first book in Braille that I read after my loss of sight, that it was not intended for people like me. I realized that sight and light were the symbols of truth and that darkness and blindness were symbols of sin and disbelief, and I realized the meaning of this symbolism in my heart, not just in my head. When, as a sighted theological student, I had written essays about the symbolism of the Fourth Gospel, I knew these things only from my scholarship, such as it was. Now I knew them from my humanity, my blind humanity, but it had not occurred to me that the Bible as a whole was written by sighted people for sighted people. I felt confused and alienated by John's Gospel, but I had not realized the reason for my reaction, because I did not know that sight and blindness generate different worlds of human experience.

When I return to your Fourth Gospel today, it is very clear to me that more than any other Gospel it is a product of a sighted society. In your presence, Lord, I read the first chapter. Verse 4 tells me that you are life, and that your life was the light of all people. Your light shines on in the darkness, and the darkness has not overcome it (v. 5). The true light (v. 9) which enlightens everyone was coming into the world. No one has ever seen God (v. 18), but we (indicating your sighted followers) beheld your glory. It is by sight that John the Baptist recognized you (vv. 33, 34). John was told that the one upon whom he saw the dove descending (v. 32) would be the chosen one, and then he adds, 'I myself have seen and have testified that this is the Son of God' (v. 34). In verse 42, we read that you looked at Peter and said, 'You are Simon son of John', and so on. Now I notice the repeated invitation to 'come and see' (vv. 39, 46). This is what you said to your disciples when they asked where you lived, and Philip said to Nathanael, 'Come and see'. When he saw you, John said to his own disciples, 'Here is the Lamb of God' (v. 29), and when you saw Nathanael coming to you, you said, 'Here is truly an Israelite' (v. 47). You said to Nathanael, 'I saw you under the fig tree' (v. 48). In the eighth chapter of this your Fourth Gospel you say that you are the light of the world and that the one who follows you will not walk in darkness but will have the light of life (v. 12); but, my Lord, I walk in darkness every day and have done so for 30 years. Yes, I know that you only meant it metaphorically, but it is not very nice to be regarded as a metaphor of sin and unbelief. Sometimes the metaphor is so graphic that I can't help feeling a twinge of pain. 'Are there not twelve hours of daylight? Those who walk during the day do not stumble, because they see the light of this world. But those who walk at night stumble, because the light is not in them' (John 11.9–10). The assumption of this passage is that work is only possible during the daylight hours, but for me the daylight hours are irrelevant. It makes no difference to me whether I work by day or by night and my computers and tape recorders, like myself, know nothing of light or darkness.

There is another question that I want to ask you, Lord. Do you believe that there is a connection between disability and sin? Or, if not you yourself, then did your early followers believe this? When you had healed the lame man who lay on the steps beside the pool of Bethesda, you said to him, 'Do not sin any more, so that nothing worse happens to you' (John 5.14). To my mind, that clearly indicates that you thought there was a connection between his lameness and some sin or other; and when I read in John 5.3 that in the portico lay a multitude of invalids, blind, lame and paralysed, I cannot imagine that this comment applied only to the particular man or to lame people in general, but would also have been said if the healed person had been blind. Similarly, when you healed the lame man lowered through the roof (Mark 2.1–12) you first said to him 'your sins are forgiven'. It was only when the implications of this comment were challenged by those who heard it that you continued with the physical healing of the lame man. It is difficult to resist the view that it was necessary first to get the sin out of the way before the disability could be healed.

FROM A BLIND DISCIPLE TO A SIGHTED SAVIOUR

When we read about the blind man in John 9 the situation is different, but presents its own problems. Your Disciples anticipated a connection between disability and sin with the question 'who sinned, this man or his parents, that he was born blind?' You rejected this suggestion, adding 'that God's works might be revealed in him' (v. 3). In other words, the man had been blind from birth not because of some parental sin but in order to create a sort of photo opportunity for you, my Lord. When you spoke of God's works being revealed in the blind man, you were not referring to his blindness, but to the restoration of his sight. The implication is that God's works cannot be seen in a blind person but only in a blind person becoming sighted.

Towards the end of the chapter we read that you said, 'I came into this world for judgement so that those who do not see may see, and those who do see may become blind' (v. 39). Some of the Pharisees near you heard this and said to you, 'Surely we are not blind, are we?' You replied, 'If you were blind, you would not have sin. But now that you say, "We see", your sin remains' (John 9.40–41). When you said 'If you were blind, you would not have sin.' this seems to mean, 'If you were really and literally blind, you would have no sin, but now that you say, "We see", your sin remains.' The sin lies not in the literal blindness but in the self-deception of those who believe that they have insight but do not.

Now, Lord, an important problem: why was there not a blind person among your followers? I know that women and black people have been asking you similar questions about themselves, but even if there were none in your group of 12, women can find models of faith in people like Mary and Martha, and there is always your mother. As for black people, they can look to representatives such as Simon from Africa, who carried your cross, and the Ethiopian traveller in the Acts of the Apostles. What models of faith do we blind people have? There is the man born blind in John 9 and there is Bartimaeus together with several unnamed people, but the trouble is that they did not become your followers until they had left their blindness behind them. This is why there was not a blind person among your Disciples and why there could not have been one: you would have restored their sight and then they would no longer be blind. Given your assumptions about blindness, which you shared with the rest of the society of your day, it could not possibly have been different. After all, if a blind person was invited to follow you and did so while remaining blind, everyone would have been shocked, and I dare say that even you would have been embarrassed. People would have said of you what they said of the Lazarus business: 'Could not he who opened the eyes of the blind man have kept this man from dying?' (John 11.37). Could not this man (that's you), who opened the eyes of other blind people, have restored the sight of your chosen follower? In terms of the assumptions of your day, it would have been difficult to find an answer to this question.

Furthermore, if a blind person could not have been your disciple in the days of your earthly ministry, what is the situation of your blind followers today? In spite of everything the theologians say about symbolism, most Christians tend to take the stories about you at face value, and a blind Christian is often made aware of the question that hangs in the air unspoken: if your faith was genuine, would not Jesus have restored your sight? I have been a member of various churches in which healing services have been held from time to time. Although they have always emphasized that healing is intended in the general sense of a blessing, not necessarily or even at all a physical restoration or regeneration, I have never felt free to attend such services, because I think that my attendance would be read in an ambiguous way. Some people might think that I was coming in expectation of the restoration of my sight. Indeed, I have known Christians who belonged to more conservative congregations who have been harassed by an expectation of miraculous healing. I have known Christians who, having become blind, have had to move to a new congregation.

You remember, Lord, the disabled people's church in South Korea which I was invited to attend. When I asked the people why they found it necessary to have their own church, they replied, 'Because the people in the ordinary churches tell us that we make them feel uncomfortable.' You and I both know of similar stories from Britain, told by blind people seeking ordin-

FROM A BLIND DISCIPLE TO A SIGHTED SAVIOUR

ation to the Christian ministry. Although many are accepted and welcomed, others are met with the objection that they would not be able to care for other people since they themselves require care. Every time one of the stories about how you restored the sight of blind people is read out in church, blind Christians will imagine the thoughts of the congregation directed towards them with the question: if it happened to Bartimaeus, why not to you? Of course, the modern miracle-working evangelists often tell stories of how you have restored the sight of blind people in their meetings. You know that because of certain experiences of my own I am slightly sceptical about these stories, but perhaps it happens. Am I not like Naaman the Syrian general who had leprosy, refusing to wash in the river Jordan because it seemed too easy? All I have to do is walk down the aisle and be humble enough to accept the ministry of healing. Perhaps, the voice of the tempter continues, it would not work for me, but I will not be any worse off than I am now.

This is the dilemma that a literal interpretation of your healing miracles has created for me, and you know that I go for comfort and strength not to the stories of your miracles, which I find alienating and distressing, but to the experience of your apostle Paul. He was given some kind of physical handicap which he called a thorn in the flesh, and there are some indications that it could have been a visual problem (1 Cor. 13.12; Gal. 4.13–15; 6.11). Anyway, he prayed three times to you, asking that it should be taken away, and you said to him, 'My grace is sufficient for you, for power is made perfect in weakness' (2 Cor. 12.8–9). Like Paul, Lord, I have no dramatic stories to tell, no accounts of wonderful happenings to amaze people with. All I have to boast of is my infirmity, my weakness.

On the other hand, you know and I know that the stories about your miraculous healings, whatever may lie behind them, have been interpreted symbolically in the Gospel traditions. For example, in Mark 8, there is a story about your healing of a blind man in two stages. At first he saw imperfectly that people looked like walking trees. After the second intervention, the man saw perfectly. This story may contain elements of folk medicine but, in the theological imagination of the evangelist, it seems very likely that it represents the limited understanding which your Disciples had in the days of your earthly ministry. It was only after the Spirit came, and the Church was formed, that a deep and true understanding of your nature and mission was achieved.[11] There are many indications in the Gospels that unbelief is spoken of as if it were a failure to see. When your Disciples did not understand you, you said to them, 'Do you have eyes, and fail to see?' (Mark 8.18), and the two disciples who walked with you on the Emmaus road after your resurrection were unable to recognize you because of their unbelief, but when you had broken the bread in their presence 'their eyes were opened' (Luke 24.31).

The negative symbolism attached to blindness runs right through the Bible. Samson, Zedekiah and Tobias were all blinded in circumstances associated with sin, folly or unbelief, and the blindness of the wicked men of Sodom (Gen. 19.11), and of Elymas the magician who obstructed the work of Paul in Cyprus (Acts 13.4–12), are specifically attributed to divine punishment. The wicked meet with darkness in the daytime, and grope at noonday as in the night (Job 5.14), the children of treacherous friends will be afflicted with blindness (Job 17.5), and the light of the wicked is darkened so that they cannot see (Job 22.11); the Psalmist complains that since God has punished him, the light of his eyes has gone from him (Ps. 38.10), and he hopes that his enemies will be cursed with blindness (Ps. 69.23); those who have been forsaken by God complain that they grope 'like those that have no eyes' (Isa. 59.10); and when the day of the Lord comes, God will bring blindness upon people, 'that they shall walk like the blind' (Zeph. 1.17).

It is this legacy of blindness regarded as a punishment from God or as a metaphor of sin and disbelief which the New Testament inherits. The most influential passage occurs after the story of the vision of Isaiah in the Temple:

> Go and say to this people: 'Keep listening, but do not comprehend; keep looking, but do not understand.' Make the

---

11 E. S. Johnson, 'Mark VIII: 22–26 The Blind Man from Bethsaida', *New Testament Studies* 25 (1978), pp. 370–83.

mind of this people dull, and stop their ears, and shut their eyes, so that they may not look with their eyes, and listen with their ears, and comprehend with their minds, and turn and be healed. (Isa. 6.9–10)

It is significant that this passage does not refer to blindness, but to the shutting of the eyes. This is a more acceptable way of describing unbelief and disobedience, because sighted people may close their eyes deliberately to avoid seeing, whereas the metaphor of blindness is not only negative towards people who really are blind but suggests that the people concerned, the sighted ones, could not help their disobedience and their unbelief. Isaiah 6.9–10 is referred to or quoted in all four Gospels, and the notion that the people have deliberately shut their eyes so as not to realize the truth of the teaching of Jesus is retained in Matthew 13.14–15 (compare Mark 4.12 and Luke 8.10). However, in John's Gospel, the metaphor of shutting the eyes is abandoned and instead the metaphor of blindness is used:

And so they could not believe, because Isaiah also said, 'he has blinded their eyes and hardened their heart, so that they might not look with their eyes, and understand with their heart and turn – and I would heal them.' (John 12.39–40)[12]

This is consistent with the emphasis in John's Gospel upon darkness and blindness as metaphors for disbelief (John 9). If any of the four evangelists had described one of your followers as being blind, it would have been a contradiction of the meaning of the symbolic universe of the ancient world as expressed in the Bible.

This negative symbolism of blindness was, of course, all too natural in a world where blind people suffered from an immense disadvantage, a world without guide dogs, white canes, Braille and computers. Nevertheless, I remain puzzled at the failure of the biblical authors to have any real insight into the lives of blind people. There is no reference to the cleverness and ingenuity of

---

12 J. M. Lieu, 'Blindness in the Johannine Tradition', *New Testament Studies* 34 (1988), pp. 83–95.

blind people, who must find different ways of doing things; there is no reference to the sensitivity of blind people to sounds and smells. Nothing is said in admiration of the intelligent hands of the blind weaver or the blind potter. True, there are references here and there to the alleged charisma and intuitive knowledge of blind people, but this is a mere illusion of sighted people who cannot resist the thought that blindness is either to be associated with outrageous sin or with wonderful wisdom.

One of the few indications of any close observation of the lives of blind people is in connection with the way that blind people walk. 'They meet with darkness in the daytime, and grope at noonday as in the night' (Job 5.14). Naturally, day and night are indistinguishable visually to totally blind people, but the reference to groping is a typical sighted person's point of view. Blind people necessarily use their hands to find things out and to protect themselves. This is not a stupid, senseless groping but an intelligent way to respond to the blind situation. A detail is added in Isaiah 59.10, where we 'grope like the blind along a wall, groping like those who have no eyes'. Yes, we blind people do make contact with the fabric, we like to keep a hand on the rail, and if we are cane-users we need something to act as a tapping board. However, this is no more than our way of glancing around, something sighted people do with their eyes, that we do with our hands, canes or with our entire body.

The impact of these observations upon sighted people is summed up in Zephaniah 1.17: 'I will bring such distress on people that they shall walk like the blind'. Blind people generally worked and lived within their families. Blind craftspeople might perhaps be seen in the marketplace, but it was not until they got up to go that their peculiarities became obvious to the sighted passers-by. Blind people do have a very visible kind of walk. You, Lord, were aware of this fascination with the way that blind people walk when you made your comment about falling into ditches.

In spite of all this, Jesus, you were not unaware of the typical sins of sighted people. If I read your Sermon on the Mount, remembering that you were a sighted person, I can appreciate it as an attack on the sighted culture to which you belonged.

> You are the light of the world. A city built on a hill cannot be hidden. No one after lighting a lamp puts it under the bushel basket, but on the lampstand, and it gives light to all in the house. In the same way, let your light shine before others, so that they may see your good works and give glory to your Father in heaven. (Matt. 5.14–16)

These sayings are obviously addressed to a sighted audience, and the visual theme is continued in verse 28: 'everyone who looks at a woman with lust has already committed adultery with her in his heart'. This is immediately followed by the warning: 'If your right eye causes you to sin, tear it out and throw it away; it is better for you to lose one of your members than for your whole body to be thrown into hell.' The eye is the instrument of adultery, so the tearing out of the eye, which makes this kind of adultery impossible, is equivalent to castration. Do not blind heterosexual men desire women? Yes, of course, but their desire is aroused through the erotic qualities of the female voice, which is inextricably bound up with the personality. The sighted heterosexual man, on the other hand, may be aroused by the sight of the female body, which in picturesque form can be disassociated from the personality. Thus the voice is erotic but the depersonalized body may be pornographic.

In Matthew 6, the attack upon the sighted culture grows stronger still. It is because of appearances, the love of being seen, that sighted people fall into hypocrisy and falsehood; but you, Lord, suggest the limits of sight when you speak paradoxically of your Heavenly Father who sees in secret (Matt. 6.5–6). That means your Father knows in a way that surpasses sight.

I particularly like the prayer you taught your Disciples, because there is nothing in it that cannot be said by a blind person. The reference to being led is particularly appropriate for blind people, and the prayer seems to suggest the superficiality and limited nature of the sighted culture (Matt. 6.9–15).

In Matthew 6.22f., you state:

> The eye is the lamp of the body. So, if your eye is healthy, your whole body will be full of light; but if your eye is unhealthy,

your whole body will be full of darkness. If then the light in you is darkness, how great is the darkness!

Not only is this a comment from a sighted prophet addressing a sighted world, but it suggests the horror and revulsion that a sighted person may feel towards blindness. Yes, indeed, the sighted world is full of show and vain glory, as you describe it when you speak of Solomon in all his glory (Matt. 6.29). People should not be bothered about their appearance or their clothing. The sighted world is preoccupied with these external things. The saying about seeing the speck which is in your brother's eye but not noticing the log in your own eye continues the theme in visual terms, speaking of the self-deception which a sighted culture encourages (Matt. 7.3–5).

Although you were a sighted person, you were not immersed uncritically in the values and attitudes of the world of sight. You were sharply aware of the temptations of vision. I also notice the restraint that you showed in your dealings with blind people. You were not at all like the modern healing evangelists, who invite disabled people to come to their meetings, and make a great show of healing them in public. I do not read that you ever encouraged blind people to approach you; rather, it was they who sought you out. A beautiful example of the tact and respect that you showed to blind people may be found in the story of the blind beggar, Bartimaeus. When he came to you, you did not assume that he wanted his sight restored but asked him, 'What do you want me to do for you?' (Mark 10.51). Now, a modern blind person would have replied, 'Get me on a good training course where I can search the internet with voice synthesizers,' but although Bartimaeus was not in a position to make this reply, it was at least nice to be asked.

When I turn to some of your other sayings, I get a better idea of your attitude towards blindness. '[W]hen you give a banquet, invite the poor, the crippled, the lame, and the blind. And you will be blessed, because they cannot repay you, for you will be repaid at the resurrection of the righteous' (Luke 14.13–14). This is part of your teaching about the reversal of status between the rich and the poor. You are to extend hospitality to the powerless. So far, I agree with you. But your message is a mixed one. You seem to take the low economic condition of blind people for granted. We are among the marginalized. We are invited to the banquet precisely because we have nothing to offer. Would my hunger overcome my fear of being patronized in this way? Are there no blind people who could be invited for their amusing conversation, or because they can play the piano while the coffee is being served? Blind people are invited because they can do nothing, offer nothing. What we have to offer is our weakness. When we are weak, the host is strong, whereas the attitude of Paul was that when he was weak, he was strong. His strength lay in his own weakness, not in the weakness of others. When you told the parable of the great feast, the idea is slightly different. The invited guests have refused to come to the banquet, because they are too busy. So the host says to his staff, 'Go out at once into the streets and lanes of the town and bring in the poor, the crippled, the blind, and the lame' (Luke 14.21). When this was done, there was still room, and the staff were told to go out 'into the roads and lanes, and compel people to come in, so that my house may be filled' (v. 23). In this story the disabled are invited not because they have nothing to offer but in order to fill the tables. They are to be included not because they are disabled but because there is room.

I have found several relevant aspects of your life and teaching. As a sighted person you seem to share the negative attitudes of your society towards blind people. At the same time, you are highly critical of the values of the sighted culture in which you live. On an individual basis you are sensitive and tactful towards blind people, and while acknowledging their condition of economic deprivation, you insist upon their inclusion. Nevertheless, you did not include a blind person in your closest circle. In your presence blind people felt the hope and discovered the reality of the restoration of sight, but you did not offer to blind people courage and acceptance in their blindness. You would have led me by the hand out of blindness, but you would not have been my companion during my blindness.

This is a cause of confusion and pain to me and many blind people, and those who have other disabilities. You accepted the fishermen. Even when they left their boats and nets on the shore, they would continue, in a sense, to be fishing. You accepted the children, embraced them, and said that they were to be models of the Kingdom. You accepted the ministry and friendship of women, even those who had a shady past, but blind people had to become sighted before they could follow you.

I am confused, Lord. I am not only hurt and puzzled; I am offended.

John the Baptist in prison sent messages to you asking if indeed you were the Messiah, or whether he should look for someone else. At that time, you cured many sick people, you cast out evil spirits, and on many who were blind you bestowed sight (Luke 7.21). Then you said to the messengers:

> Go and tell John what you have seen and heard: the blind receive their sight, the lame walk, the lepers are cleansed, the deaf hear, the dead are raised, the poor have good news brought to them. And blessed is anyone who takes no offence at me. (Luke 7.22)

This answer is intended to reassure John the Baptist, and we must presume that John would have been offended if you had not been restoring sight to the blind. My position is just the opposite of his. I am offended because you did restore sight to the blind, although I am very happy for the individuals who were thus restored. What I want is inner healing, the healing that comes from acceptance, from inclusion, from the breaking down of barriers through mutual understanding, for an acceptance of different worlds, of different kinds of human life. You seem to present a convergent model of normality but I want a divergent model. This is why I am offended.

Nevertheless, your word comes home to me as it did to John in prison. I am also to be blessed if I am not offended by you, but how can I help being offended?

Your evangelist Matthew applies to you the prophecy of Isaiah. You were healing many disabled people, and Matthew says that this was in fulfilment of the prophecy, 'He took our infirmities and bore our diseases' (Isa. 53.4 and Matt. 8.17). But to perform miracles upon disabled people is not to take their infirmities and to bear their diseases; it is to remove them. There is a difference between taking something away and taking something upon yourself.

As I read your Gospels, thinking about these problems, I come upon a passage which I have known all my life, but it has never struck me before how relevant it is to my present life as a blind person. After they had tried and sentenced you to be condemned to death, the servants of the High Priest began to spit on you, blindfold you and strike you, saying 'Prophesy!' (Mark 14.65). Luke describes the incident as follows:

> Now the men who were holding Jesus began to mock him and beat him; they also blindfolded him and kept asking him, 'Prophesy! Who is it that struck you?' They kept heaping many other insults on him. (Luke 22.63–65)

To be blindfolded is not to be blind. To be a sighted person who cannot see is not the same as to be a blind person. Nevertheless, it begins to come close to it. In these moments of *de facto* blindness, did you begin to know blindness from the inside? Did those words come back to you – 'blind fools'? Now you yourself are treated like a blind fool. Strangely, my indignation begins to die away. My questions are silenced. You have become a partner in my world, one who shares my condition, my blind brother.

Later in the same day, they crucified you. From about midday, there was darkness over all the land. It was then that you cried out, 'My God, my God, why have you forsaken me?' (Mark 15.34). In your agony and confusion, did you realize that there was an eclipse of the sun? Or did you think that once again they had blindfolded you? Or that perhaps you had indeed lost the power of sight? Was that perhaps why you felt forsaken by God, the God of light, the sighted people's God? I cannot help wondering whether, after these experiences, your attitude to blindness is somehow different. On the road to Emmaus, the eyes of your two disciples were constrained, so that they were not able to recognize you (Luke 24.16). You walked the road with two disciples who were in effect blind. Only when you broke the bread were their eyes opened so that they could recognize you, and then you vanished from their sight (Luke 24.31). Again, they became blind as far as you were concerned, but now it is the blindness of recognition, no longer the blindness of a failure to recognize. Sight has become more paradoxical.

The Gospel of John foresees the end of the sighted culture. 'I am going to the Father and you will see me no longer'; and, later in the same chapter, 'A little while, and you will no longer see me, and again a little while, and you will see me' (John 16.10, 16). This awareness of the limits of sight is vividly expressed in the story of Thomas, who doubted your resurrection. You said to Thomas, 'Have you believed because you have seen me? Blessed are those who have not seen and yet have come to believe' (John 20.29). Most people think you were speaking to second and third generation Christians, or those living far away from Israel, who never saw your earthly ministry. However, these words can be regarded as a particular blessing upon your blind disciples.

When I began to write to you, my mind was full of questions. Then my confusion turned into indignation; and then I wrote with tears when I realized that you not only died for me but you became blind for me. And what can I say to you now about the passages that offended and hurt me so much? Well, Lord, if I may say so without presumption, I forgive you. But is it not your role to forgive me? Yes, but perhaps our relationship is becoming more mutual. Blind people, after all, do lead other blind people. You have been this way before, so you are familiar with it. Take my hand, blind master, and lead me.

Yours sincerely
John

Implications for the Education of Both Blind and Sighted People

The attitudes of people in our culture towards blindness are shaped by the classical literature of western society, reinforced by repetition in many novels and films.[13] This cultural construct is further reinforced by the metaphorical use of blindness in everyday speech.[14]

This inherited set of attitudes and beliefs is ambivalent towards blindness. On the one hand, blind people are thought of as helpless, pathetic, useless, ignorant, or even stupid, insensitive and incompetent. On the other hand, blind people are sometimes regarded as being strangely gifted. They have amazing memories and may have a weird kind of foresight. Blind people are regarded with a mixture of admiration, compassion and horror. A sighted person, sharing these attitudes towards blindness, who loses his or her sight transfers inwardly all of the previous images and presuppositions about blindness.[15] The blinded person now has feelings of horror and compassion towards the self. All the helplessness and ignorance that were imputed to other blind people now recoil upon the self. Thus blindness is a shattering blow to one's self-esteem. This is reinforced by the attitudes of compassion and horror with which the blind person is now greeted by relatives, friends and, above all, employers. The blinded person comes quickly to agree that he or she might get hurt, will have to retire and is no good at anything any more.

---

13 Eleftheria A. Bernidaki-Aldous, *Blindness in a Culture of Light*, Frankfurt: Peter Lang, 1990; William R. Paulson, *Enlightenment, Romanticism and the Blind in France*, Princeton: Princeton University Press, 1987; D. Kent, 'Shackled Imagination – Literary Illusions about Blindness', *Journal of Visual Impairment & Blindness* 83:3 (1989), pp. 145–50.

14 The COBUILD Bank of English held in the University of Birmingham contained more than 750 examples of the word 'blind' from the pages of the *Guardian* newspaper on 23 October 1998. Of these, only 45 per cent are literal. In all but one or two cases, the remaining metaphorical uses are negative towards blindness: 13 per cent emphasize blindness as ignorance, 12 per cent as deliberate indifference, 28 per cent as culpable ignorance (often severe and violent), and 0.02 per cent refer to callous indifference. The remaining 15 per cent are miscellaneous negative expressions. We read of 'blind and insensitive planning', 'blind blithering arrogance', and 'sheer blind obsessiveness'. What use does the word 'blind' serve in these expressions? None, except for providing the satisfaction of using as an expletive a human condition the name of which happens to begin with the letter b. These comments are not a criticism of the *Guardian*. On the contrary, if a socially aware newspaper such as this expresses the negative image so vigorously, we may assume it to be used with less sensitivity elsewhere.

15 A. Wagner-Lam and G. W. Oliver, 'Folklore of Blindness', *Journal of Visual Impairment & Blindness* 88:3 (1994), pp. 367–76.

Of course, the shock of blindness is very great, since it is necessary for the personality to reconstruct itself around a different balance of the senses, and the reluctance to exchange one world for another is as profound as the reluctance to lose sight in the first place.[16] Nevertheless, these elements of change in the inner and outer worlds of blindness are certainly accentuated and complicated by social attitudes towards blindness, built up over the centuries.

Since the Bible has been the principal source of cultural definition in Europe, it is not surprising that it is also the principal source of the cultural construct of blindness.

The attitude of Jesus towards blindness has been the inspiration for the medical and social care of blind people in Europe and beyond.[17] The fact that blind people were the objects of the healing ministry of Jesus, and that the recovery of sight was one of the main features of the coming of the Kingdom of God, has undoubtedly led to improved conditions for blind people.[18] At the same time, however, the negative images of the Bible have also been significant. While the miraculous healing of blind people is obvious, external and memorable, the negative images of blindness in the Bible are subtle, often metaphorical, and almost unnoticeable. The fact that the reader of the Bible is immersed within the cultural construct of blindness largely created by the Bible means that the attitudes towards blindness in the Bible are hardly noticed even as they are read. There is no contrast between the construct of blindness in the Bible and that which is prevalent in our society. As one reads the Bible, the attitudes in the Bible towards blindness are, so to speak, camouflaged by the lack of contrast between them and what we think about blindness anyway. Thus what takes place is an uncon-

---

16 Maurice Merleau-Ponty, *Phenomenology of Perception*, London: Routledge and Kegan Paul, 1962, pp. 81f.

17 It is significant that prophets and evangelists have often sought to establish their credentials by healing or attempting to heal blind people. An example is the attempt of the millenarian prophet Richard Brothers to heal the blind in 1788. See J. F. C. Harrison, *The Second Coming: Popular Millenarianism, 1780–1850*, London: Routledge and Kegan Paul, 1979.

18 Gabriel Farrell, *The Story of Blindness*, London: Oxford University Press, 1956, p. 150; Paulson, *Enlightenment*, p. 8.

scious process of reinforcement. We read the Bible in the light of our cultural construct of blindness, which is at the same time replicated and reinforced by what we read.

One might suppose that the moment one goes blind the truth of this collaboration in prejudice would become apparent. One might imagine that a blind person reading the Bible would quickly detect the disparaging identification of blindness with ignorance, unbelief and sin, but recognition and identification seldom take place with such immediacy and such simplicity. The blind person does not recognize the images any more than the sighted person does, and, rather than pointing to the Bible as the source of the oppression, the blind reader points to himself or herself as the person described in the Bible. The blind person reads that Jesus called sighted people blind fools. The blind person, especially the blind religious person, does not usually think that Jesus should not have used such language because blind people are not necessarily fools. On the contrary, the blind Christian simply accepts what Jesus said.

The educational implications of this situation for both blind and sighted people are far-reaching. It is essential to develop a critical metaphorical awareness of the biblical text, which is contrary to the literalness too often preferred by the devotional reader of the Bible.

This attitude towards blindness has been constructed not only by the Bible but by the self-enclosure of sighted people. It can be deconstructed by helping sighted people not to be enclosed within their sighted world. This can be attempted through helping both blind and sighted people to realize their own unconscious constructs. The techniques of personal construct psychology such as the pyramid grid are useful ways of doing this.[19] Next, these constructs, having been brought to the surface, can be placed against the images and presuppositions of the Bible. This involves a deconstruction of the cultural artefact through which we read the Bible, and also at a deeper level a reconstruction of the cultural artefact of the sighted world out of which the Bible came in the first place.

---

19 Alvin Landfield and Franz R. Epting, *Personal Construct Psychology, Clinical and Personality Assessment*, London: Human Sciences Press, 1986.

The Christian education of blind and sighted people in particular, and of so-called able-bodied and disabled people in more general terms, is very much in need of such a liberating pedagogy. As a result of such a process, blind people, whether religious or not, will be able to live with more self-respect and self-understanding. If sighted people can learn to adapt to the needs of blind people without patronizing them, and if blind people can learn to accept sighted people without manipulating them, the new relationship of mutual acceptance between blind and sighted will have become a utopian whisper of a new world.

Implications for a Theology of Blindness

At a conference where I had spoken about a biblical theology of blindness, I was the object of a very funny satire which was presented to the members of the conference during a concert on the final evening. My good-natured critic, much to the amusement of everyone, proposed a theology of baldness, which would be inspired by my approach. He presented several passages from the Bible which suggested a prejudice against bald people. The bald Samson was a weak Samson; the boys ridiculed Elisha by shouting out 'Get out, you bald head!', and in general hair is regarded as an ornament and crowning beauty, hence to be without hair was to be dehumanized and ugly.

This clever parody made me re-examine my view of blindness. By identifying in detail the particular characteristics of one condition or another, we begin to grasp the fact that some human conditions are so radically different that they create different worlds.[20] A *state* of human life is a condition sufficiently distinct from others, and sufficiently radical, to create its own world. Being a child is such a state, and male and female are also such states. A theology of blindness, or of any other major disability, may then be thought of as a theology of the states of life. Its

---

20 An outstanding medical psychologist whose detailed observations have helped us to realize the character of these human states is Oliver Sacks. See especially his *Awakenings*, London: Duckworth, 1973; *A Leg to Stand On*, London: Duckworth, 1984; and *Seeing Voices: A Journey into the World of the Deaf*, London: Picador, 1991.

theological antecedent may be found in the seventeenth-century French school of mysticism associated with Pierre Bérulle.[21] The human states are not so foreign to each other that mutual understanding is impossible, but on the other hand they are sufficiently distinct to create real challenges to self-enclosure. Such states are generated through a combination of physical and social characteristics, and the balance between the physical and the social may well vary. Skin colour can produce such states, and in societies which are acutely conscious of pigmentation there can be more than a dozen distinct social groups, each identified by a different skin colour.[22] However radical the different experience of life is for black and white people, this difference is the product of imperialism and has no secure ground in physiology as such. Speaking purely psychologically, black and white people may experience life in very much the same sort of way. That is not true of childhood, since although childhood is very largely a cultural artefact,[23] there are necessary biological and developmental factors which would constitute childhood as a distinct state no matter what the character of the cultural construct.

The difference between a state and a non-state will be a matter of criteria which will be arranged along a continuum. Blindness is undoubtedly a state of human life, since blind people live in a world of experience which is radically different from that in which sighted people live.[24] The same may be said, perhaps even more emphatically, of the world of the profoundly deaf person. Adults who do not grow taller than three foot six have

---

21 A state is a feature of the life or being of Jesus which is 'concrete, permanent and independent of powers and actions, imprinted in the depths of the created being and in the condition of its state'; Henri Brémond, *A Literary History of Religious Thought in France*, Vol. III. *The Triumph of Mysticism*, London: SPCK, 1936, p. 56. States are 'modes of being'; see Eugene A. Walsh, *The Priesthood in the Writings of the French School*, Washington, DC: Catholic University of America Press, 1949, p. 7.

22 In Haiti, pigmentations may be significant by a ratio of 127:1 parts white to black. In other words, if a person has one black ancestor seven generations earlier, he or she can be categorized accordingly; Thomas H. Eriksen, *Ethnicity and Nationalism: Anthropological Perspectives*, London: Pluto, 1993, pp. 63f.

23 Philippe Ariès, *Centuries of Childhood*, London: Cape, 1962.

24 I have explored this theme in some detail in *On Sight and Insight: A Journey into the World of Blindness*, Oxford: One World, 1997.

an experience of adult life which is so radically different that this condition may be said to be world-creating; but to be a bit on the short side is not the same. It is a sliding scale. In a society of equal opportunities between men and women, the degree to which gender is a world-generating state will be somewhat minimized, although never entirely absent; but in societies where there is rigid gender stereotyping, the world of women may be very different from that of men.[25]

Baldness is not a world-creating condition in our society. It is an attribute of a world but not a world. It may be regarded as a loss, perhaps an embarrassment, and if it is the result of a loss of hair following chemotherapy, baldness could be a cause of acute distress. Nevertheless, it remains a distressing feature of the sufferer's ordinary world, and does not throw him or her into the sort of reconstruction of reality which is necessitated by becoming paralysed from the neck down, for example.

A theology of blindness is an example of what might be called a theology of states or conditions. It is similar to and yet different from feminist and black theologies. Like them, it will have both negative and positive aspects; it will both denounce and announce.[26] A theology of blindness will try to expose and denounce the negative imagery that flows from the sighted world,[27] and it will at the same time try to relativize the taken-for-granted assumption of the sighted world that the sighted reality is absolute. Being sighted is also a state.

Next, a theology of blindness will be constructive. It will propose that blind people reflect the image of God in their very blindness. It will show that the metaphor of blindness suggests in a positive way the essential characteristics of the life of faith. From a theology of blindness we can derive practical sugges-

---

25 John Gledhill, *Power and Its Disguises, Anthropological Perspectives on Politics*, London: Pluto, 1994, pp. 34–8.

26 Paulo Freire, *The Pedagogy of the Oppressed*, London: Sheed and Ward, 1972, p. 76 and *The Politics of Education*, London: Macmillan, 1985, p. 57.

27 Many examples could be provided to illustrate the negative image that blindness has in the Christian theological tradition. The sermon 'Christ the Light of the World' by Jonathan Edwards (1703–58) is full of negative images of blindness. Wilson Kimnack (ed.), *Jonathan Edwards: Sermons and Discourses 1720–23*, New Haven: Yale University Press, 1992, pp. 535ff.

tions about social and political life. These might include the techniques of taking one step at a time, and concentrating on the concrete particularities of an otherwise overwhelmingly abstract problem. A theology of blindness, like any theology of disability, will challenge prevailing concepts about what is normal. The traditional view is that when the Kingdom of God comes, the eyes of the blind will be opened, the ears of the deaf will be unstopped, and the lame person will jump like a deer. A theology of blindness will show that, instead of contemplating utopia in terms of a convergence upon a single image of normality, what we must converge upon is a wider acceptance of varieties as being normal.[28] Normality must become inclusive. This will lead us into a critique of other forms of exclusion, including the most powerful of all, the exclusion of the poor by the rich. In some such way, a theology of blindness will offer a utopian promise of universal liberation.[29]

---

28 Jane Wallman, 'Disability as Hermeneutic: Towards a Theology of Community', unpublished Ph.D. thesis, University of Birmingham School of Education, 2000; for other recent writings on theology and disability, see Judith Z. Abrams, *Judaism and Disability*, Washington, DC: Gallandet University Press, 1998 and David A. Pailin, *A Gentle Touch: From a Theology of Handicap to a Theology of Human Being*, London: SPCK, 1992; and for a recent philosophical treatment Bryan Magee and Martin Milligan, *On Blindness: Letters Between Bryan Magee and Martin Milligan*, Oxford Oxford University Press, 1995.

29 I have tried to suggest the utopian symbolism of blindness in the postscripts of *On Sight and Insight*, pp. 233f.

5

Blindness and the Face of God

Toward a Theology of Disability

God as Above Average

The human image of God is usually thought of as the image of the perfectly normal human, but raised to an even higher level of perfection. God never sleeps. '[H]e who keeps you will not slumber. He who keeps Israel will neither slumber nor sleep' (Ps. 121.3b–4). God could not be thought of as suffering from upper limb malfunction or as being hard of hearing. 'See, the LORD's hand is not too short to save, nor his ear too dull to hear' (Isa. 59.1). The God who is in the image of the perfect human being must possess all the faculties and members of perfect humanity. 'He who planted the ear, does he not hear? He who formed the eye, does he not see?' (Ps. 94.9). God is thought of not only as a sighted person, but as a person whose sight far extends the power of human vision. 'For the LORD does not see as mortals see; they look on the outward appearance, but the LORD looks on the heart' (1 Sam. 16.7). 'Sheol is naked before God, and Abaddon has no covering' (Job 26.6). When God made human beings in God's own image, inference from the normal human body suggests that God must have the normal human powers when thought of in human terms. God walks in the Garden of Eden; God does not limp (Gen. 3.8). 'Ascribe to the LORD, O heavenly beings, ascribe to the LORD glory and strength' (Ps. 29.1). If God is to have a voice, the voice of God must be louder than the voice of the mighty warriors. 'The voice of the LORD is powerful; the voice of the LORD is full of majesty. The voice of the LORD breaks the cedars' (Ps. 29.4f.).

The God of the Bible is the God of the able-bodied not of the disabled. Women were not permitted to be priests (Lev. 21.16–20), and the God of the Bible is not a woman. Men with a physical defect were not permitted to be priests, and the God of the Bible does not possess physical defects.

No doubt all this is obvious and was inevitable. Indeed, that the image of God is a projection from able-bodied life is so obvious as to be generally invisible by the able-bodied. After all, sighted people do not know that they are sighted. They think the world is just like that. The world of sight is absolutized as being the only world. This sighted world must be relativized if minority groups are not to be marginalized. The biblical image of God in human likeness represents the domination of the normal, the totalism of the average.

Such language is not a mere poetic decoration. It is not to be understood on the linguistic level, as if it were a mere case of metaphor, and to classify it as anthropomorphism is inadequate, since that would be to gather up the whole of humanity within the average. The form (*morphe*) of the human (*anthropos*) is thought of as comprising only the normal. The human family, however, extends beyond the normal; it comprises many who are not average. If the word were poly-anthropomorphism, the plurality of the human forms would be affirmed, but the fact is that the human image of God in the Bible is not many-formed but is uniform.

There are signs of weakness, of course. God weeps, has changes of mind, proceeds by trial and error, and suffers parental disappointment (Gen 2.18f.; 6.6; Hos. 11.1f.), but all this is still within the range of the normal. If the God of the Bible suffers from parental disappointment and failure, it is because God's children are rebellious and disobedient, not because God cannot strike them hard enough to maintain discipline, or cannot run fast enough to catch them. We must go deeper than the levels of metaphor and analogy if we are to understand the nature of these projections. The metaphors are but symptoms of a certain kind of embodied epistemology.

Body-Knowledge

Much modern semantic theory regards meaning as residing in propositions. Only propositions are capable of carrying meaning, which may be true or false in accordance with its successful reference to the actual world. This leads to the possibility of a universal language in which reality is objectively described. The world of truth and the propositions that embody truth is distinct from the worlds of imagination and memory, which are regarded as being individualistic. As sensations or perceptions, such individual experiences are not capable of contributing to the positive or negative character of truth unless they can be stated in linguistic form. On this objectivist view of language, truth is to be found in the relationship between symbols, these in turn being spoken or printed words built into sentences. Although empirical verificationalist forms of this semantic theory insist that the meaning of propositions must be translatable in principle into certain experiences or sensations, the body is looked upon as the locus for the verification of meaning rather than being regarded as the source or origin of meaning itself.

This rejection of the body as the source of meaning is consistent with objectivist views of theological language. According to such views, religious or theological meaning is also found in sentences which express beliefs. Those who defend the truth-claims of religious statements against positivistic semantics usually do so by qualifying or denying the empirical verification theory, but share with their opponents the view that bodily experiences are not relevant to the search for truth. Truth resides in ideas or beliefs. Truth, it is thought, is spiritual or intellectual. Truth is stated in concepts, which are interrogated by the rational mind, to which the body makes no contribution.

Thus the flesh is to be distinguished from the spirit. The flesh and the spirit are antagonistic to each other. The body is the source of fantasies, desires, impulses, imaginations and temptations, which far from helping us to discover the truth must continually be checked and corrected.

In seeking to understand the human image of God as a contribution to a theology of disability, we must commence not with the formal belief structure of Christian theology, which exists as ideas, beliefs and concepts in the form of sentences, but with an epistemology rooted in bodily structures. To be disabled is to have a different physical or mental structure. It is these structures themselves which must be the starting point for a theology of disability, and this can only be done if the body itself becomes the starting point for knowledge, and thus for understanding the human image of God.

The question we must ask, therefore, deals not so much with the nature and criteria for knowledge, but with the character and origins of understanding. When we ask about how we understand, the human questions about memory, cognition, expectation, self-deception and so on inevitably arise. Mark Johnson has pointed out that statements of human knowledge would be incomprehensible without their metaphorical content.[1]

'We will have to find a *way* around the problem.' 'The next *step* in the argument is as follows.' 'Let us have a *closer look* at this question.' The metaphors in sentences such as these are not merely decorative, nor do they merely tend to make our conversation more colourful. Rather, Johnson argues, they may be traced back to patterns of experience or schemata, in which our bodily experience is generalized. Without such fundamental experiences, which occur from earliest infancy, of distinguishing between this and that, of being in front or at the back, of going forward or being blocked, of learning about place and weight and time and so on, it would not be possible for us to make our lives in the world intelligible. Our language is the fruit of these deep roots, and thus our thinking is embodied right from the start.

This does not lead Johnson into a wholly subjective theory of meaning, for the basic bodily experiences are common to all human beings, and most of them are developed in social relations. This is why the metaphors that express bodily experiences linguistically are confirmed in public life, and bodily knowledge, notwithstanding its individual origin, remains public. Knowledge

---

[1] Mark Johnson, *The Body in the Mind: The Bodily Basis of Meaning, Imagination, and Reason*, Chicago: University of Chicago Press, 1987.

is thus produced by a combination of subjective and objective factors. It is both bodily and conceptual, situational and yet universal. This is what Johnson means by a 'semantics of understanding'.[2]

Bodies and Words

Johnson's main concern is to establish the epistemological significance of imagination, and he does this through describing the roots of imagination in physical and social experience. In his understandable concern to defend his theory of imagination from the charge of excessive subjectivity, he emphasizes the shared nature of metaphorical experience, thus establishing a degree of objectivity for the imagination. In this context, he does not distinguish between different kinds of bodies. So although his work is valuable as an epistemological introduction to a phenomenology and a theology of disability, he does not take us into that specific area.

This is less true of the phenomenological philosophers and psychologists upon whom Johnson depends. Maurice Merleau-Ponty provides the heading 'The Body' for the first part of his *Phenomenology of Perception*.[3] My body is my point of view upon the world. My body is the perspective from which I perceive everything else, but I forget this.[4] Instead, I come to regard my body as just one more of those things that I perceive to be in the world. Then I speak as if on the table are my book, the telephone and my hand. I situate my body in space just like the other things in the space around me. Merleau-Ponty remarks that this is misleading, since the other objects in my world may sometimes be present and at other times absent, but my body is always there. The body is not itself an object in the world; it is that by means of which, for me, there are objects. A theory of the body is thus already a theory of knowledge. However, because

---

2 Johnson, *Body in the Mind*, p. 175.
3 Maurice Merleau-Ponty, *Phenomenology of Perception*, London: Routledge and Kegan Paul, 1962, p. 67.
4 Merleau-Ponty, *Phenomenology*, p. 70.

what is known is dependent upon the conditions of knowledge, we become unaware of the creative intentionality of our own consciousness.

Merleau-Ponty illustrates this world-generating character of embodied knowledge by referring to the world as known by various kinds of unusual bodies. He discusses the white cane of the blind person, pointing out that, as the hand of the blind person holds the cane, the hand is not aware of the cane itself, but of the ground surface as revealed by the cane.[5] The sharp point of consciousness moves forward from the grip of the hand down to the tip of the cane. In other words, the cane becomes an extension of one's body.

The experience of the phantom limb reported by patients who have suffered amputation is particularly significant. The foot itches although it has been removed. We should understand this strange phenomenon not in terms of neurological conditioning – for example, your brain has always been used to receiving sensations from that part of your body and it goes on regardless – but should instead interpret the phantom limb as representing the acceptance on the part of the entire body of living in a certain world. The body has a certain way of relating to that world. The refusal to acknowledge dismemberment is a way of insisting upon remaining in that world.[6] One represses the knowledge that one's body can no longer be at home in that world. If one accepts the mutilated body, then one's world becomes fractured. The task of building up a new world as a new relationship between the dismembered body and the world is more painful and challenging than the other option: preserving one's normal world and denying dismemberment.

The visual parallel to this is Anton's Syndrome, which takes place when patients are unaware of their own blindness. They behave as if they can see and even confabulate visual experiences.[7] When this condition is generalized to include the denial of any impairment or disability, it is called *anosognosia*. Sometimes a

---

5 Merleau-Ponty, *Phenomenology*, p. 143.
6 Merleau-Ponty, *Phenomenology*, p. 81.
7 Andrew W. Young, *Face and Mind*, Oxford: Oxford University Press, 1998, p. 380.

patient with a double impairment is aware of one but not of the other.[8] I acknowledge that my world is fractured in this respect but not in that respect.

We may distinguish phenomenal consciousness from access consciousness. Phenomenal consciousness means that I am aware of realities. Access consciousness means that I know that I have this awareness of realities. The object of phenomenal consciousness is the world itself, but the objects of access consciousness are symbols, words and thoughts. This distinction is well established in the experimental literature, where people deny that they have seen the flashing of a light but can point to the area from which the light flashed. 'Studies of blindsight strongly suggest that the processing of visual stimuli can take place even when there is no phenomenal awareness of seeing them.'[9] In other words, information can be obtained from visual areas in spite of the fact that there is no conscious visual awareness. Amnesiac patients who are shown a range of pictures may later on be unable to remember that they have been shown the pictures or even taken part in such an experiment, but may be able to distinguish between pictures that are familiar to them and those that are not. There appears in such cases to be phenomenal memory without access memory.[10] A sleepwalker who safely negotiates a window ledge has phenomenal consciousness but no access consciousness.

These cases of malfunction are relevant to the general phenomenon of world projection from the body. Gender is a case in point. Gender so thoroughly permeates my perceptions and interpretations of myself and of the world that it becomes invisible to me. As a man, I may become unaware of my masculinity; to me, that is just the way things are. My phenomenal awareness is so taken for granted as the basis of my experience that I do not possess access awareness of it. It is the task of gender training which combats sexism to raise phenomenal awareness to the level of access awareness. We can now understand why it is that most sighted people do not know that they are sighted but just think the world is like that. They have phenomenal aware-

---

8 Young, *Face and Mind*, pp. 379f.
9 Young, *Face and Mind*, p. 375.
10 Young, *Face and Mind*, pp. 379f.

ness of sight but little access awareness of it. Only when the clock stops ticking do you realize that you have been hearing it. Only when you become blind do you realize that you were living in a sighted world. So it is that most sighted people, who have perhaps never experienced disability or had occasion to empathize with a disabled loved one, do not acknowledge a plurality of genuine human worlds. To them, there is the common-sense world to which some people do not have access. Thus there is the world of normality and there are disabled people who have the misfortune to be excluded from that world. Relativization is the key to pluralization, and pluralization is the key to mutual understanding and acceptance.

The Face of God in the Bible

Nowhere is this monism of the majority more obvious than in the biblical references to the face of God. 'When he [God] is quiet, who can condemn? When he hides his face, who can behold him?' (Job 34.29). 'They think in their heart, "God has forgotten, he has hidden his face, he will never see it"' (Ps. 10.11). 'As for me, I shall behold your face in righteousness; when I awake I shall be satisfied, beholding your likeness' (Ps.17.15). 'May God be gracious to us and bless us and make his face to shine upon us' (Ps.67.1). 'So Jacob called the place Peniel, saying, "For I have seen God face to face, and yet my life is preserved"' (Gen. 32.30). When Jacob had become reconciled to his brother Esau, he said, 'for truly to see your face is like seeing the face of God – since you have received me with such favour' (Gen. 33.10).

These and many other similar passages reflect a sighted person's view of the world, including relationships with other human beings. The projection from the human face to the face of God is particularly clear in the way Jacob addresses Esau. Not only is this perfectly natural; it is almost impossible to imagine that it could have been otherwise. However, when the unconscious and taken-for-granted preference for the world of the sighted person is accompanied by an equally unconscious but all-pervasive prejudice against the world of blind people, we have an ethical problem, a problem of inclusion, a problem of the absolutization of the normal to the exclusion and disadvantage of the minority. Throughout the Bible blindness is a symbol of ignorance, sin and unbelief. We find this metaphorical use as early as Exodus 23.8: 'You shall take no bribe, for a bribe blinds the officials and subverts the cause of those who are in the right' (cf. Deut. 16.18–20). 'Israel's sentinels are blind, they are all without knowledge; they are all silent dogs that cannot bark' (Isa. 56.10) 'Let them alone; they are blind guides' (Matt. 15.14). Blindness is generally regarded as a punishment inflicted by God (Gen. 19.11; Deut. 28.27–29; 2 Kings 6.18; Acts 13.10–12).

It is the references in the Gospels to blindness that display most vividly the prejudices of the sighted world and are the cause of most distress to blind people. The healings of blind people are generally regarded as symbolic of discipleship.[11] This is particularly clear in the story of Bartimaeus (Mark 10.46–52). As a result of his faith, he followed Jesus along the way (v. 52).[12] The symbol of blindness as unbelief and sin occupies the central place in the Gospel of John,[13] where the discussion at the end of chapter 9, following the restoration of sight to the man born blind, reveals this clearly: 'Jesus said, "I came into this world for judgement so that those who do not see may see, and those who do see may become blind"' (v. 39).

Some of the most vivid passages in which the sight of the human face is used as a symbol of spiritual progress and enlightenment appear in the letters of Paul. 'For now we see in a mirror, dimly, but then we will see face to face' (1 Cor. 13.12); 'And all of us, with unveiled faces, seeing the glory of the Lord as though reflected in a mirror, are being transformed into the same image from one degree of glory to another' (2 Cor. 3.18); and, perhaps the most beautiful and significant of all such passages, 'For it is the God who said, "Let light shine out of darkness", who has

---

[11] E. S. Johnson, 'Mark VII: 22–26: the Blind Man from Bethsaida', *New Testament Studies* 25 (1979), pp. 370–83.

[12] E. S. Johnson, 'Mark X: 46–52: Blind Bartimaeus', *Catholic Biblical Quarterly* 40 (1978), pp. 191–204.

[13] J. M. Lieu, 'Blindness in the Johannine Tradition', *New Testament Studies* 34 (1988), pp. 83–95.

shone in our hearts to give the light of the knowledge of the glory of God in the face of Jesus Christ' (2 Cor. 4.6).[14]

Living Without Faces

What does the human face mean to a blind person? At this point, I must speak rather personally, but I know that other blind people share my experience. In the months that followed my own loss of sight, I began to notice that the people of my acquaintance fell into one of two possible groups. There were those who had faces, when I conjured up their image in my memory, and there were those who did not have faces. The first group were those whom I had known before I went blind; the second group were those people whom I had met since my loss of sight.[15] At first, I could not help imagining what these people might look like, and vivid impressions of various facial appearances would flash before my imagination.[16] Gradually, however, as I entered more deeply into the blind condition, the vivid imaginations faded. After some years, I had reached the point where I was so naturalized into the world of blindness that it was only with a slight shock of surprise that I could remember that people looked like anything. I had not only lost the images of the faces of particular people; I had lost the entire category of looking like anything. I had to make an effort of memory to realize that to sighted people there was something called 'look like' which was very important to them.

No doubt it is difficult to imagine the world in which other people live. If you, as a sighted person, were to close your eyes, and think of one of your dear friends or loved ones, the picture of the face of that person would irresistibly come to mind. Try it now, and see if you can prevent the image of the face appearing in your imagination. Some of the sighted people I have asked tell

---

14 I have attempted to respond as a blind person to the Bible in my *In the Beginning There Was Darkness: A Blind Person's Conversations with the Bible*, London: SCM Press, 2001 and Harrisburg: Trinity Press International, 2002.

15 John M. Hull, *On Sight and Insight: A Journey into the World of Blindness*, Oxford: Oneworld, 1997, pp. 14–15.

16 Hull, *On Sight and Insight*, pp. 15–19.

me that they can manage this feat for a few moments by concentrating on the shoes of the friend or by imagining that they are staring hard at a button or at the handbag which the friend is carrying. However, this seems to be difficult if not impossible to maintain: the face keeps coming into view. For a blind person, on the other hand, there simply is no face. Nothing comes into mind of a pictorial nature which represents the features of the face. The memories that a blind person has of someone else gather first around the name of the person and then around the memories of everything which that person has said and done. In the presence of the other, it is the voice that expresses the person, not the face.

One must also remember that although the senses are unified in subjectivity, the experience offered by one sense is incommensurable with another. One may tell a person blind from birth that the colour red is like the sound of a trumpet, and although this will convey the notion that redness is bold and challenging, it will not actually convey the slightest impression of redness itself. If you are my close friend, I may, perhaps, be invited to touch your face. This, however, will give me very little information about what your face looks like. Certainly, I will learn that you have a beard, but I do not remember what a beard looks like; I only know that it is short and bristly. This is most true in the case of the eyes. In the first place, it is difficult to touch the human eye. Even if you close your eyes and invite me to feel the roundness of your closed eyelid, it bears no resemblance at all to the radiant colour and fleeting emotion and the sense of inter-personal subjectivity that sighted people get through eye contact.[17]

What does the Bible know of this experience? Very little, if anything at all. Particularly in the Psalms, God is described as hiding his face from Israel. This makes sense to sighted people, for they refuse to have eye contact with people from whom they are estranged, and to look away is a gesture of dismissal, if not contempt. In the world of sighted people, you cover your face in order to disguise your identity. So the bank robber wears a

---

17 Hull, *On Sight and Insight*, pp. 47–8.

mask, and so do the people at a fancy dress party. A blind person, on the other hand, does not know whether your face is masked or not, although your voice may sound muffled. Blind people can certainly tell when you are looking at them, because your voice is projected directly towards them. It is the voice to which they pay attention, not the face.

The Bible, however, comes from a sighted world in which it was natural to speak of the human image of God in terms of the appearance of God as prefigured in the relationships that sighted people have with each other. In this context, the face is of supreme importance. 'If we are born alone, it is through the face that we first experience things out there that are like us, that respond to us, and which by making faces we can influence.'[18] 'The sharing of life and of experience, which is the joy of parenthood, begins in the face.'[19] The evolution of consciousness is difficult to understand without the face, for the face is the main access to the mind. We are biologically prepared from birth to respond to facial expression. Infants only a few days old are capable of imitating adult expression.[20] Although facial expressions might convey slightly different emotions from culture to culture, the way these emotions are recognized in, for example, movements of the eyebrows or the mouth retain their significance across cultures.[21] Experiments with computerized facial images, where either the sound of the voice or the picture of the face could be omitted or varied, show that the content of a message is better understood when the face is visible. 'In face to face communication, perception of speech does not necessarily result from just the sound but somehow emerges from the sound and sight of the face collectively.'[22]

Of course, blindness is not the only human condition that introduces a variation on the theme of the face. People with autism are not cut off from the sight of the face but are profoundly severed from the emotions and the mind behind the

---

18 Jonathan Cole, *About Face*, Cambridge, MA: MIT Press, 1998, p. 111.
19 Cole, *About Face*, p. 111.
20 Dominic W. Massaro, *Perceiving Talking Faces: From Speech Perception to a Behavioural Principle*, Cambridge, MA: MIT Press, 1998, p. 204.
21 Massaro, *Perceiving Talking Faces*, pp. 229–30.
22 Massaro, *Perceiving Talking Faces*, p. 236.

face. 'Autistic subjects actively avoid the face, to avoid complex signals of mood in other people, which on the one hand, they can hardly decipher and, on the other threaten to overwhelm them.'[23] Jonathan Cole interviewed people with many different kinds of facial loss or disfigurement and concluded that it is the world of the autistic person rather than the world of the blind that is really a world without faces, because there is no theory of mind, the mind of the non-autistic person. The only glimmering of understanding into others on the part of an autistic person is into another person with autism.[24] Mention should also be made of *prosopagnosia*, a condition in which people are unable to recognize the faces of their loved ones or friends. A remarkable feature of this strange condition is that the prosopagnosic patient can often recognize various features of the face, such as the gender, age or hair colouring, but is unable to identify the possessor of the face.[25]

In his remarkable book about the face, Jonathan Cole says that he could have interviewed film stars or well-known politicians, people whose beautiful or famous faces are always before the public eye. However, in order to probe the meaning of the human face, he decided to go to those who had in some sense lost the face, whose faces had become immobile, disfigured, palsied or blinded, and among these people he had discovered a revitalization of deep life.[26]

The Face in Philosophy and Theology

It is surprising, perhaps, that on the whole those who write books on theology and the philosophy of religion do not follow the method of Jonathan Cole. When they seek to describe human responsibility and human relationships, using the face as the focus of their writing, they assume the sole reality of the sighted world. This becomes almost ironic when the subject of

---

23 Cole, *About Face*, p. 4.
24 Cole, *About Face*, p. 197.
25 Young, *Face and Mind*, p. 378.
26 Cole, *About Face*, pp. 181f.

discussion is the miracles of the New Testament in which Jesus is described as restoring the sight of the blind. In approximately 20 such articles written in recent years, I have not found a single concession to the fact that these stories express a sighted point of view, nor any awareness of how the stories might strike a blind reader.[27] No doubt there are plenty of articles written about the healing miracles of Jesus that do display such sensitivity; it just happens that I have not come upon them.

The role of the human face is particularly noteworthy in the writings of Emmanuel Levinas. Transcendence breaks into our lives when we take responsibility for our fellow human beings, and 'such a responsibility is a response to the imperative of gratuitous love which comes to me from the face of another'.[28] The abandonment of being into existence, and the unique election of each individual, is viewed in the face. It is the face of the other that summons me to this responsibility. For Levinas, the nakedness of the face represents the vulnerability of each human being, for whom there is no defence or covering.[29] The core of the infinite is 'a summons which comes to me from the face of the neighbour',[30] 'here I am: under your gaze, obliged to you'.[31] When I relate to another, 'it is not the knowledge of his character, or his social position or his needs but his nudity as the needy one, the destitution inscribed upon his face. It is his face as destitution which asks me as responsible, and by which his needs can only count for me.'[32] Yes, but all this presupposes that one can see the face of the other.

It is clear from what has been said about Levinas that his use of the human face, although very individual and concrete, referring as it does to my presence before the specific other who claims my response, remains a symbol. Levinas is not interested in the psychology or physiology of the face. He seldom refers to the face as having any characteristics, except that the eyes of

---

27 Hull, *In the Beginning*.
28 Emmanuel Levinas, *Of God Who Comes to Mind*, Stanford: Stanford University Press, 1998, p. ix.
29 Levinas, *Of God*, p. 12.
30 Levinas, *Of God*, p. 73.
31 Levinas, *Of God*, p. 75.
32 Levinas, *Of God*, p. 99.

the other gaze upon one. For Levinas, the face does not smile or frown, it is not a face with a specific gender, nor is it a singing face. In that sense, the use of the face in Levinas is quite similar to its use in the Bible. The face of God indicates the presence of God. Nevertheless, everything depends upon being able to see the face, and the fact that Levinas so often emphasizes the muteness of the face of the other heightens the visual presuppositions of his style.

In the case of David Ford, although the symbolic character of the face becomes more apparent as his book *Self and Salvation* proceeds, the much more detailed descriptions of the face suggest a deeper involvement in the particularities of sighted life. The opening sentence of the first chapter is, 'We live before the faces of others.'[33] 'Words have their primary context in faces.'[34] The Christian Church might be described as 'the transformation of facing before the face of Christ'.

> Christianity is characterized by the simplicity and the complexity of facing: being faced by God, embodied in the face of Christ; turning to face Jesus Christ ... being members of a community of the face; seeing the face of God reflected in creation and especially in each human face, with all the faces in our heart related to the presence of the face of Christ; having an ethic of gentleness ... towards each face ...[35]

In this opening chapter, we are presented with an unrelieved visual theology. To be 'faceless' is to be anonymous, to be a non-person. Although rich and beautiful in its descriptions of the face, there is no relativization of facial experience.

This does not mean that David Ford is not sensitive towards the other senses. Chapter 5 deals with the singing self, and shows a rich sensitivity to music and to sound in general. However, even here the significance of singing lies very largely in its face-to-face character. 'Singing is seen as a desirable form of face-to-face

---

33 David F. Ford, *Self and Salvation: Being Transformed*, Cambridge: Cambridge University Press, 1999, p. 17.
34 Ford, *Self and Salvation*, p. 22.
35 Ford, *Self and Salvation*, pp. 24f.

address between members of the community, and between singers and God.'[36] 'I sing before the faces of those before whom I have learned to worship, and whom I call to worship.'[37] There are no references to deafness.

The discussion by David Ford of the face of the dead Christ is both tender and profound. We are led dramatically into the realization of the dead face. After Christ's speaking from the cross, breathing, and crying out, we are left with the sight of the dead face.[38] This, however, is surely the projection of a sighted theology. From a blind perspective, when the breathing and crying have stopped, there is nothing but silence. It is as if there is only sighted normality: the sighted normalities of life, suffering and death. Ford emphasizes with a fine theological insight that the death was a real death, and that the resurrection was a rising from the dead, not just a delayed coming down from the cross. Always, however, the face is seen.

Conclusion

Does it matter? Must majorities always take minorities into account? Cannot sighted people enjoy their world, theologize about their world, speak to each other in that world without blind people nipping their heels? After all, the principal source of Christian theology, the Bible, acknowledges blindness, deafness and other disabilities only to marginalize and denigrate them.

It matters because such attitudes reinforce the central core of Christian exclusivism. Even in the writings of such enlightened and insightful sighted people as those I have been discussing, such attitudes lend support to the core of that exclusivism which, among other things, ignores other religions, only grudgingly comes to accept the ministry of women, and supports an ideology of uniqueness and of the normality of the superior which has brought disgrace upon the Christian tradition throughout the world. It matters because in this world of approximately

---

36 Ford, *Self and Salvation*, p. 110.
37 Ford, *Self and Salvation*, p. 128.
38 Ford, *Self and Salvation*, p. 192.

three billion people, there are about six hundred million disabled people, and the gospel is for them also.

Strangely, there is one aspect of the face of Christ which Ford does not refer to. It is the blindfolded Christ (Mark 14.65 and Luke 22.64). The dead face of Christ witnesses to the laying down of his life in the nothingness of death. The blindfolded face represents the living Christ who enters into the experience of literally blinded people, and becomes their brother. While sighted people may quite naturally behold the glory of God in the face of Jesus Christ, blind people may just as naturally respond to the glory of God in the face of the one who was blindfolded for us.

6

A Spirituality of Disability

The Christian Heritage as Both Problem and Potential

Preview and Summary

On the basis of a phenomenological epistemology, according to which human knowledge is projected from the human body, spiritual development is here regarded as the transcendence and transfiguration of the body as a biological organism. The transfiguration and resurrection of Jesus Christ authorize and illustrate this view of spiritual development within the Christian tradition. This view of knowledge as embodied enables us to interpret disability as epistemologically creative. The blind body knows and lives in a blind world; the deaf body a deaf world. Each human world has its own distinctive characteristics and its own limited autonomy. The human worlds relate to each other along a continuum because, although different bodies generate different worlds, there is only one human species.

The criteria of transcendence and transfiguration also apply to the spiritual development of disabled people, although in each case relative to the characteristics of the body which is disabled, transcended, and transfigured. This enables us to conceive of a multiplicity of known and lived human worlds.

This has two advantages. First, the plurality of the human worlds enables us to construct a spirituality of disability which is not based upon a theory of deficiency. As long as the disabilities are mainly understood as lacking something, their intrinsic character as worlds will be overlooked, and they will be understood as mere exclusions from the big world. This view of disability challenges the unconscious hegemony of the average, the majority, and thus opposes all ideologies of domination, whether or not they are aware of their power.

Second, this view of the spirituality of disability extends our understanding of humanity itself by denying exclusive humanity to the majority and insisting upon the genuinely human character of the disabled worlds. In this way, humanity is enriched through variety. Plurality is richer than uniformity, and the different human worlds need each other to achieve full humanness.

Although the Christian tradition may be thought of as supporting this view of spirituality, the Bible does not endorse a plurality of human worlds but depicts a single ideal humanity which fell away into various kinds of alleged imperfection and abnormality. The Bible story tells us that these will be overcome when the perfectly human is restored. Jesus, who according to this world history is perfect humanity, is hailed as the messianic agent for the restoration of perfect and uniform humanity.

Thus the question arises as to whether we should look upon the Christian tradition as a problem rather than a potential. The truth is that elements of both problem and potential may be found in the Bible and in the various theological doctrines. A first attempt to explore this ambiguity may be to list the elements on one side and on the other.

The Nature of Spirituality

Human spirituality is that which transfigures and transcends the biology of the human.[1] When we speak of transcending the biological, we refer to those potentials of the human being which enable him or her to make the biological organism instrumental to non-biological purposes. These potentials include abstract thought, imagination, empathy, the ability to represent biological experiences symbolically, and the capacity to integrate experience and knowledge around a significance or a meaning

---

1 John M. Hull, 'Spirituality, Religion, Faith: Mapping the Territory', *Youth and Policy: The Journal of Critical Analysis* 65 (1999), pp. 45–59; John M. Hull, 'Spiritual Development: Interpretations and Applications', *British Journal of Religious Education* 24:3 (2002), pp. 171–82.

that goes beyond the pleasure and pain of the individual. Language and money are the two finest achievements of the human tendency towards the spiritual because, being relational in their character, they articulate and facilitate the experience of solidarity with other people.[2] The capacity of the human will to become integrated with others, or to dominate others as the case may be, is incarnate in money and in language.

When we speak of spirituality as transfiguring the biological, we refer to the fact that the biological is never left behind by transcendence. The body is not the antithesis of the spiritual but its organ. We should not contrast the spiritual with the material, nor should we regard the spiritual and the biological as being on altogether different levels. Rather, we should speak of transfiguration: the material infused with the spiritual, the body becoming the form of inter-subjectivity.[3]

In the Christian faith, the typical representation of spirituality is to be found in the story of the transfiguration of Jesus (Mark 9.2–8). The body was not left behind but shone with radiance. This could not occur to an isolated body, but only in the context of others, and of the speech that links person to person. This is why Jesus is seen on the Mount of Transfiguration with Moses and Elijah, and they are speaking with each other (v. 4). Even the resurrection does not leave his body behind (Luke 24.39; John 20.6f.), and, with the ascension, the transfigured body is raised to universality (Acts 1.9). The ascension into heaven of the prophet Elijah (2 Kings 2.11), the figure of the resurrected Christ (John 20.27), and the bodily assumption of Mary all indicate that the Christian faith confesses a biological spirituality, and believes in the resurrection of the body as the fulfilment of human potential (Rom. 8.23; 1 Cor. 15.42; Phil. 3.21).

---

[2] John M. Hull, 'Christian Education in a Capitalist Society: Money and God', in David Ford and Dennis L. Stamps (eds), *Essentials of Christian Community: Essays in Honour of Daniel W. Hardy*, Edinburgh: T&T Clark, 1996, pp. 241–52. See also John M. Hull, 'A Christian Perspective on Spiritual Education, Religion and the Money Culture', in James C. Conroy (ed.), *Catholic Education – Inside Out/Outside*, Dublin: Veritas, 1999, pp. 285–301.

[3] John M. Hull, *Utopian Whispers: Moral, Religious and Spiritual Values in Schools*, Norwich: Religious, Multicultural, Personal and Social Education, 1998, pp. 63–9.

Nevertheless, the body is transcended as well as transfigured. This takes place when the body of the other person is valued like my own body, felt like my own body, and even loved as my own body (Eph. 5.28). The body that is not transcended remains encircled within the membrane of the skin. Egocentricity is the enclosed body. The senses, although they appear to open the body out upon the world, do not do so unless they are met by the answering sense of the other. In the reciprocity of eye contact, or skin contact, or conversational contact, we transcend the biological nature which is transfigured in the process.

The Disabled Body and Its World

If we agree that spirituality should be regarded as that which transfigures and transcends the body, the way is open for a consideration of the epistemological implications of such an embodied spirituality. Recent work in the philosophy of phenomenology and in the philosophical implications of brain research have illuminated the body as the origin and main determinate of our knowledge.[4] The world we know is the world as projected by our bodies.

If someone is born into a disabled condition, the world generated by that state is formed from the earliest days. One is, so to speak, born a citizen of that world. On the other hand, if one becomes disabled at a later stage, whether during childhood or in adult life, one experiences the shock of losing one's world. The tendency is for resistance, and then for a terrible sense of loss, and then the disabled body shrinks back into itself. One becomes extremely conscious of having an impaired body, whether it is merely a broken arm or leg,[5] or the loss of the power of speech following a stroke, or the loss of mobility after an accident. It is then true that, whereas most people live in the world, dis-

---

[4] Maurice Merleau-Ponty, *The Visible and the Invisible*, ed. Claude le Fort, Chicago: Northwestern University Press, 1968; Mark Johnson, *The Body in the Mind: The Bodily Basis of Meaning, Imagination and Reason*, London: University of Chicago Press, 1987; Georg Lakoff and Mark Johnson, *Philosophy in the Flesh*, New York: Basic Books, 1999.

[5] Oliver Sacks, *A Leg to Stand On*, London: Duckworth, 1984.

abled people live in their bodies. Not only is this the result of the shock of losing the native world, but it may be particularly acute following sensory deprivation, because the normal knowledge which one had of the world has now shrunk into the body itself. The person recently blinded becomes very aware of internal body sensations.

It is at this point that the recently disabled person either renounces the old world and accepts the new, now disabled, body, or on the other hand refuses to let the old world go, insists on continuing to try to live within it, and perhaps longs and prays for the miracle which will restore not just the former body but the former world. The painful choice is made more poignant by the fact that, since the everyday world of the average person is not conscious of its distinctive character as a world but imagines itself to be the only reality, the newly disabled person cannot imagine any other world than the one he or she has now left. The normal world regards the disabled person as banished, excluded, deprived, as it were, of citizenship rights, and as therefore to be pitied and helped.

As the recently disabled person recovers from the shock of the fractured and now lost world, a new world gradually begins to dawn. In the case of a blind person, this is the world of touch, smell and hearing which, although at first disintegrated by the loss of the unifying power of sight, gradually link up with each other again. The body regroups, consciousness reforms itself, and a new world appears. In the case of the person who has lost hearing, a new experience of living within vision appears,[6] and communication becomes focused on the hands. The body builds up its new world, relating to it with new powers and functions for different parts of the body. In the case of the blind person, the hands are no longer mainly used to do things, but now to know things and finally to appreciate beauty.

As the new world is gradually built up, put into place with innumerable fits and starts, the disabled person is no longer confined to the broken body, but begins again to inhabit a world. No longer merely an exile, he or she applies for and is granted

---

6 Oliver Sacks, *Seeing Voices: A Journey into the World of the Deaf*, London: Picador, 1991.

citizenship of a new place. The body is again integrated within its world, and the former world remains as a dream, an occasional flash of regret, a pang perhaps, only to be overtaken by the intrinsic meaning of the new world within which one must not only exist but live.

The process of world formation may be thought of as transfiguring the body, since the person now extends from the body into which life had at first shrunk, and feels its way out again. Under certain circumstances, and for certain persons, the disabled body may be not only transfigured but transcended. One sometimes finds oneself forgetting that one is, in the opinion of the old world, disabled. Needless to say, access to the new information technology is an enormous boon to many disabled people, opening up for them again a world of knowledge and communication that transcends the limits of their disabled bodies, just as it transcends the limits of any body.[7]

In this way, we may begin to speak of a spirituality of disability, the spirituality that transfigures and then transcends the body, while springing from it and remaining united with it, a spirituality made all the more powerful, in some cases, by the fact that it is created as an achievement whereas the world into which one was originally born was always taken for granted. The spiritualized disabled person has been born again, with fresh awareness of the world, and of the plurality of worlds. No longer confined through the deception of everyday experience within an absolute world, the spiritualized disabled person finds, often to his or her surprise, that life is enjoyed at a deeper level.

Many Bodies, Many Worlds

The transfiguration of disability reveals itself as global. This means that the disabled body projects a world that is as distinctive and as autonomous as other worlds, although perhaps not

---

7 I note in particular the outstanding work of AbilityNet, the principal voluntary organization in the UK for providing computer advice and assistance for people with disabilities. For information, consult www.abilitynet.co.uk or contact AbilityNet, PO Box 94, Warwick, CV34 5WS.

as independent, in view of the fact that the world of the normal or average is by far the most powerful.

One of the most important aspects of the spirituality of disability lies in the challenge that it offers to hegemony. The world of the able-bodied usually conceives of itself as the only world. Those whose bodies are not able are excluded. As an example, let us take the situation of sighted people. Although sighted people know, with varying degrees, that they are sighted, it is unusual to find a sighted person who knows that he or she lives within a world that is a projection of the sighted body. In other words, although sighted people know that they know through sight, they seldom realize the epistemic implications of vision.[8] Sight projects a world and sighted people are embodied within that world. They know that there are others but they seldom know that there are other worlds. Therefore they think of others as being excluded from their own world. Thus they unconsciously create a discourse of dominance.

When this ideology of domination is internalized by disabled people, as is almost inevitable in the first instance, the result is a loss of self-esteem, a loss of soul which is the accompaniment of identification with the marginalized and the excluded. In this way, the power of the present absolute world is acknowledged.

There can be no dialogue between the disabled and the non-disabled until the plurality of human worlds is recognized. As long as the non-disabled world retains its hegemony, the relations that it has with the world of disability will be those of care for the helpless, and of patronization. The relationship will be that of charity, of condescension, and not that of mutual respect based upon acknowledgement of otherness.

However, once it is recognized that the apparently single world must be pluralized, then the relative breaks down the absolute. The absolute is incapable of dialogue. In the relations between able and disabled people, that is significant but perhaps not central for the future of our species. However, once the hegemony of the single world in the relation between able and disabled people is broken, a challenge is mounted against all

---

8 Maurice Merleau-Ponty, *Phenomenology of Perception*, London: Routledge and Kegan Paul, 1962.

other human worlds that claim to be absolute. The world of the globalized market which claims to be the only way forward for the world is challenged by other possible human futures.⁹ The world of absolute religious truth is likewise challenged to give way to multiplicity. Disability offers us a way of dialogue, and so the spirituality of disability becomes politically significant. Inside the money-curtain, the communities of disability have the potential to become subversive elements, while outside the money-curtain disabled communities bear witness to the sufferings of a dehumanized humanity, colonies within colonies, the marginalized within the marginalized, the frontier of the human, where Christ dwells.

Disability and the Widening of the Human

We have seen that a spirituality of disability makes a contribution to the wider spirituality of the human by breaking down the absolute world of the powerful. There is a second aspect to this: a spirituality of disability helps us to gain a wider concept of the human itself.

If the body were to be thought of as having an immediate capacity to represent and symbolize the mind, the spirit, or the character, then the disabled body would indicate a disabled mind, a tortured face would indicate a tortured spirit, a blind body would indicate spiritual blindness.[10] Any spirituality which the disabled body might have would be but a remnant, a fractured representation of a higher and more perfect spirituality; but now the transfigured body is no longer only the body of the athlete transfigured through motion and skill, or only the body of the dancer transfigured through the beauty of rhythm and form, but includes the broken body transfigured towards otherness and self-transcendence. This is because the pain of the body, and the social marginalization of the body which is differ-

---

9 Susan George and Fabrizio Sabelli, *Faith and Credit: The World Bank's Secular Empire*, London: Penguin, 1994; Ulrich Duchrow, *Alternatives to Global Capitalism*, Utrecht: International Books, 1995.

10 Joanne Finkelstein, *The Fashioned Self*, Oxford: Polity Press, 1991.

ent from that of others, can lead the transfigured disabled body into an identification with a more comprehensive bodily range, whereas the body of the athlete or the dancer is caught up into the transfiguring beauty of skill and motion but does not in itself imply or demand sympathetic identification with a range of bodily experiences. If the variety of human bodies is thought of as being arranged in the form of a pyramid, social values would place the beautiful, skilful body at the apex; but it is at the base that most area is covered, where the most comprehensive variety of bodies is understood. The transfigured disabled person knows the variety of human conditions and thus has an opening into other worlds. Emptiness understands fullness in a way that fullness cannot understand emptiness. It is true that the empty desires the full, and the full fears the empty, but in its transfigured state the broken body may learn to be beyond desire and fear.

Because disabled people are socially defined as those who are not average, not normal, but disabled, no longer abled, they are necessarily sidelined, marginalized, pigeon-holed, stereotyped. They themselves, however, have the capacity to transfigure the broken body, the marginalized body, into a symbol of inclusion through sacralizing the extremities of humanity. It is the very provinciality of disability that enables it to grasp the territory of the human, while the city, looking out upon the provinces, thinks that it itself is everything.

So a spirituality of disability not only pluralizes the human world, but extends it.

The Christian Tradition

Although the Christian tradition faces both ways in the struggle between the rich and the poor,[11] the powerful and the powerless, it certainly does not face both ways in the struggle between the hegemony of the single world and the plurality of the human worlds. On the contrary, the Bible is almost unequivocal in

---
11 Ernst Bloch, *Atheism in Christianity: The Religion of the Exodus and the Kingdom*, New York: Herder & Herder, 1972, p. 25.

expressing the point of view of the able world. God is portrayed as an able-bodied God.[12] God has powers of sight beyond the normal, powers of knowledge beyond the average. God is super-abled. It is inconceivable that God should be a disabled God. 'See the LORD's hand is not too short to save, nor his ear too dull to hear' (Isa. 59.1). The result is a humanity of convergence, where the signs of redemption are to be found in the recall of the peripheries to the centre. 'Then the lame shall leap like a deer, and the tongue of the speechless sing for joy' (Isa. 35.6). This convergent humanization is modelled upon the perfection of the creation, in which everything reproduces according to its kind (Gen. 1.24f.), so assuring the stability and continuation of the characteristics of normality. The convergence is rooted in the domination of the majority and returns in eschatological visions towards the singularity of the average.

Jesus is the archetype of this normality, without spot or blemish (1 Pet. 1.19) and without deviation from the image of God which is the normal (Heb. 1.3). He takes little children in his arms (Mark 10.16), accepts the caresses of working women (Luke 7.38), and touches the outcast (Mark 1.41). He recognizes the spiritual authenticity of those who lie outside the orthodoxies of Judaism (Luke 7.9) and recognizes that those who do the will of God in all nations are his brothers and sisters (Mark 3.35). Only the disabled seem incapable of inclusion within this universal realm of accepting love. We see the force of this if we ask the naïve question why there were not disabled people among the group of close disciples of Jesus. There were none, and it would have been impossible that there should have been any, for the simple reason that Jesus would have restored such people to full health. Indeed, such restoration becomes in itself symbolic of the experience of becoming a disciple. The blind Bartimaeus sits beside the road begging but the sighted Bartimaeus follows Jesus in the way (Mark 10.52). The struggle of Jesus against disability is his contest with the powers of Satan (Luke 13.16). As eschatological Son of Man he actualizes the convergence of which the

---

12 See Chapter 5 of this book.

prophets spoke (Matt. 8.17), and as magical healer he brings the disabled out of the power of darkness (Luke 11.20).

Yet he himself becomes blinded (Mark 14.65; Luke 22.64), immobilized (Mark 15.24), and marginalized (Gal. 3.13; Heb. 13.12). At first he accepts the infirmities of humanity by healing them, but finally he accepts the infirmities of humanity by participating in them, by becoming one of them. 'He was despised and rejected by others; a man of suffering and acquainted with infirmity' (Isa. 53.3).

The Christian Tradition and Disabled People

Jesus the miracle worker, the one who did not have disabled people among his Disciples, is the Jesus who has lived on most powerfully in the Church.[13] Since blindness was a symbol of sin and unbelief, it has continued to represent stubbornness, ignorance and insensitivity. The charismatic healers down the centuries have had the satisfaction of knowing that whenever they tried to heal blind people they were involved in the mission against Satan, and Jesus who exorcised the powers of evil was seen as blessing the work of every evangelist who tried to drive out the blind demons.

This has had consequences for both good and evil as far as disabled people are concerned. In the first place, it has meant that blind people have been cared for by those who believed that they were imitating Christ in doing so. The literal nature of this imitation of Christ can be seen in the fact that Christian missions tended to be more active towards the various diseases and infirmities that were the object of the healing of Jesus. To heal the blind, the deaf, and those who had leprosy was obviously to imitate Christ; Christian missions towards those who have diseases not mentioned in the Gospels have not been quite so prolific. On the other hand, granted the social conditions, it was better that blind people should receive compassion and care than that they should starve. However, there was an alternative policy that depended upon making a distinction between disease

---

13 See Chapter 4 of this book.

and disability, between those who were sick within a certain world and those who lived in other human worlds. This would have meant accepting plural forms of humanity, and this would have meant qualifying or abandoning the biblical discourse of exclusion, in which the myth of a perfect creation leading to a perfect restoration would have been abandoned. It would have meant accepting disabled people into ordinary congregational life, and this would not have found an ideal model in the Gospels unless Jesus had had disabled people among his Disciples; and, given the conditions of that day and the symbolic meaning of disability to which the Gospel writers were committed, that would have been impossible. I must refer to my experience with a church for disabled people to which I was invited. They told me that they found it necessary to meet together because the people in the ordinary churches felt uncomfortable in their presence.

There were two alternatives confronting the Christian movement. One option was represented by the healing of blind Bartimaeus, and the other by the blindfolded Christ. In one tradition the removal of blindness becomes an allegory of entering into the Christian life; in the other tradition blindness itself is made sacred by the presence of Christ within it. In the first tradition a rhetoric that disparages blind people becomes essential to the discourse of salvation; in the other possibility the treasure of redemption is carried around in 'clay jars' (2 Cor. 4.7). In one tradition the glory of God is seen when a blind person becomes a sighted person (John 9.3); in the other possibility, the grace of God is experienced in weakness (2 Cor. 12.9).

Paul saw it all very clearly. The way of love is preferable to the way of miracles (1 Cor. 12.31). The plurality of bodily parts is preferable to the domination of the uniform (1 Cor. 12.12). The thorn in the flesh is a greater witness to the grace of God than the heavenly religious experience (2 Cor. 12.1–9). In the four Gospels blindness is symbolic of lack of faith; but in the letters of Paul and in Hebrews it is faith that is blind (Rom. 8.24; 2 Cor. 5.7; Heb. 11.1).

The ambiguity of the rhetoric in which blindness may sometimes stand for sin and sometimes for the achievement of faith is not of mere literary or even theological interest. It is a question of the identity of blind people and of how the Church is to regard them. This itself is indicative of the wider issue of disability: how disabled people are to achieve identity and how society is to grant them an accepted and honoured place. At an earlier point in our discussion, the rhetoric of wholeness which drew its strength from the disparagement of disability seemed to be so overwhelming in the pages of the Bible that it was unclear how the Bible could even be thought of as being on both sides of this conundrum. All the power seemed to lie on the able side. Now that we have considered the matter more deeply, it is clear that there is ambiguity, but it has been suppressed beneath the power of uniformity. Why did it take two thousand years for the Bible to be identified as a book written by sighted people?[14] Why did it take so long to recognize that the sighted people's Bible has excluded blind people? It is because uniformity goes with centrality, with authority, and with power. The anti-disabilist rhetoric of the powerful Church grew side by side with, and for the same reasons as, the anti-Semitic discourse. Disabled people and Gypsies participated with Jews in the Holocaust. In the dichotomized world-view of the seventeenth century, of which the twentieth century was the inheritor, the world was divided between white people and the others, Christians and others, the male and the female, the body and the deviant body.

Christian Faith as Problem and Possibility

One of the problems for a theology of disability, which would speak in a Christian way about the spirituality of disability, lies in the fact that almost all theological authors, being themselves sighted people, write unconsciously from a sighted perspective which has the effect of emotionally and symbolically excluding blind people. I think that the same is true of people with

---

14 John M. Hull, *In the Beginning There Was Darkness: A Blind Person's Conversations with the Bible,* London: SCM Press, 2001 and Harrisburg: Trinity Press International, 2002. This, as far as I know, is the first attempt to interpret the Bible from a blind person's point of view.

other disabilities, particularly those who do not have normal hearing, but blindness is the only example of which I have intimate knowledge. An example would be the continued use of the symbol of the face to represent human relationships, and to represent the presence of God. Theologians and philosophers who do this, whether Jewish or Christian, are guided by the biblical imagery of the face of God, which represents the presence of God. However, in writing like this it is all too easy to overlook the fact that the human experience of the face differs widely. Not only are there faces that are conventionally beautiful or ugly, but there are many diseases of the face, people unable to move the facial muscles, and people who have suffered terrible deformations of the face because of injuries and accidents. There are mental conditions that make it impossible for people to recognize the human face, and there are blind people, who can touch the face but cannot see it and for whom the experience of the face is profoundly different.[15] To touch a pair of smiling lips is not the same as being smiled at. This unconscious hegemony of the sighted is an instance of an ideology of dominance, and it must be questioned, if the Christian faith is to be genuinely open to all sorts and conditions of people.

The Christian tradition also includes positive elements which could be developed into a theology of disability. These include:

1 the blindfolded Christ;
2 the general picture of Christ as suffering and as being immobilized and identified with the abnormal, the cursed;
3 the theology of incarnation in which God accepts a body, leading us to believe that it is through the body that our faith should be matured;
4 the incarnation as an indication of emptying, of God's acceptance of vulnerability, of the abandonment of the divine perfection (Phil. 2.5–8);[16]
5 the theology of the heavenly session in which Christ shows his wounds to the Father in intercession for humanity. This

---

15 Jonathan Cole, *About Face*, London: MIT Press, 1998.
16 Nancy L. Eiesland, *The Disabled God: Toward a Liberatory Theology of Disablity*, Nashville: Abingdon Press, 1994.

indicates that the body of the ascended Christ is not a perfect body, but a body of scars (Heb. 7.25);
6 the theology of Saint Paul and the Letter to the Hebrews in which sightlessness becomes a symbol of faith;
7 the experience of Paul in discovering that the strength of God was perfect in his own experience of disability;
8 the varieties of gifts given to the Church, which suggest a rejection of the monolithic body in favour of the variegated body;
9 the plural theology in which many worlds are recognized, God being the Lord of all worlds.

Educational Implications

The concept of spirituality as being an inter-subjective elevation of the biological leading a person beyond self-centredness into solidarity with others, when applied to disabled people, suggests a spirituality of various human worlds. The advantage of this is that it enables us to take each other seriously in whatsoever state or condition we may be, and prevents us from looking upon any member of the human family as worthless or as a human deviant. The educational significance of this is that to understand disability does not require compassion, let alone pity, but it does demand that one should be able to enter into a world very different from one's own. One must learn to see the way the other worlds look from within the world that one has entered. This might be done through studying the poetry written by quadriplegics, attending the Paralympics, reading the literature of pathography. Another educational approach would be by means of denunciation. One could gather examples of the use of expressions like 'blind' and 'dumb' to indicate a state of sin in, for example, a typical hymnbook.[17] Examples of the use of disparaging metaphors based upon various disabilities could be gathered from the newspapers. Yet another approach might be to heighten awareness of the senses through the temporary elimination of one sense. The easiest sense to suspend is sight,

---

17 See Chapter 9 of this book.

but the experience of being forbidden to speak for a day or spending a day in a wheelchair can be just as enlightening.

What are the implications of this approach for the education of disabled children and adults? One of the controversies within special education is the question of whether disabled children should be educated for successful life in the larger society or whether they should be educated for successful life within the world they already live in. This controversy was particularly sharp in the case of those with profound hearing loss, and has only gradually been partially resolved in a deeper respect for the integrity of the deaf condition and the recognition that the culture of the visual has its own characteristics.[18] In the history of the education of people with a visual loss, there has been a similar conflict.[19] The predominance of embossed, punctilinear script over embossed shapes of the letters of the Latin alphabet is a case in point. Punctilinear script, the most widespread example of which is the type devised by Louis Braille, is recognizable by touch more easily than the embossed forms of printed letters, but is less convenient for sighted people. Braille only won the struggle when blind people got control of the agencies. The approach of this present study is a contribution to the growing tendency to recognize the integrity and distinctive nature of each form of disability, and lays emphasis upon the need to help each disabled child to achieve wholeness within the characteristics of that particular disabled state. For social and economic reasons, disabled people must also live in the greater world, but this can be achieved most successfully if the adaptation to the larger society springs not from a sense of deficiency and loss but from a position that has come to realize the intrinsic character of the world in which one lives in the body.

I realized this in the course of preparing my project 'Cathedrals through Touch and Hearing', which set out to equip the English cathedrals with facilities for blind and partially sighted visitors. I found that most of the cathedral guides wanted to show the sighted person's cathedral to the blind person and did

---

18 Sacks, *Seeing Voices*.
19 Pamela Lorimer, *Reading by Touch: Trials, Battles and Discoveries*, Baltimore, MD: National Federation for the Blind, 2000.

not understand that such knowledge must necessarily remain in words only. How can a blind person be interested in stained glass? Only by way of general information about the cathedral. Sighted guides would place the tip of my finger on a tiny rose bud, cleverly carved among the intricate shapes of the leaves and branches of a chair leg, something that would take the blind hand a long time to appreciate, while the loveliness to the hand of the cold brass of the smooth communion rail would not be mentioned. Gradually my project team realized that blind people must be taught to acquire first-hand knowledge of the cathedral, and this meant teaching them to use their bodies in contact with the fabric in order to construct a distinctive blind cathedral. We realized that there are at least two cathedrals – one for sighted and the other for blind people. Each has its beauties and its needs.

This approach is also significant for Christian education within the churches. Not only is it a step towards a more inclusive congregation, but the challenge to the able-bodied hegemony requires a new way of interpreting the Bible and the hymnbooks, and this in turn suggests new directions for Christian spirituality. The restrictions placed on personal development when people remain in a literal, one-dimensional stage is removed when the unacceptable consequences of biblical literalism are exposed. The problem of the relation between the first chapter of Genesis and contemporary science can perhaps be resolved without abandoning literalism, but how can the biblical negativity towards disabled people be maintained? The challenge to the moral authority of the Bible suggested by a theology of disability is more difficult to resolve, and new understandings of the spirituality of the Bible are demanded.

Is there any hope of the success of this enterprise? Is not the prejudice against disabled people so ingrained in our religious tradition and so unconsciously reinforced week by week by readings from Scripture and in the singing of many traditional hymns that there can be little chance of new attitudes emerging? Perhaps this is so, but attitudes do change, and the unconscious prejudice of today may become the deliberate bias of tomorrow, and with this greater awareness there is hope of reform. Change is taking place more rapidly in the world than in the Church, so once again let the world write the agenda, and life inside the churches may also change.

Conclusions

We have seen that there is a natural spirituality of disability which points to the variety of human bodies and human experiences as making up the whole human world, and that this poses a challenge to the structures of unequivocal power that rule our world. We have also seen that to some extent the Christian faith produces and collaborates with this hegemony of power. We have also seen from the rich variety of its ambiguity that the disabilist theologian may be able to recover elements that may form the basis for a theology of disability. Such a theology will link with a spirituality of disability in the sense that it will give specific religious articulation to the natural, experienced spirituality of the various conditions of disabled people, as each learns how to transfigure and transcend the limits of his or her biology. The position outlined in this article is not without its own ambiguity. One would not expect doctors to give up the fight against disease on the grounds that it is good to encourage a variety of human worlds, nor would we expect an ophthalmologist not to do his or her best to save someone's sight because of his or her respect for the blind world. The concept of an epistemological world is not intended to avoid the varieties of human suffering, but to honour the distinctiveness of the experience of those who permanently reside in various states. Let us hope that the Christian faith which has always motivated its adherents towards the alleviation of suffering will prove equally effective in motivating Christians to recognize variety and to challenge the concentrations of exclusive power.

7

Is Blindness a World?

From Theology of Impairment to Theology of Disability

A theology of disability must begin with the distinction between impairment and disability. Impairment refers to a physical or psychological attribute of an individual such that the individual differs in some significant respect from the normal or average person, while disability refers to the social consequences of having an impairment.[1] Impairment is sometimes referred to as the medical model of disability, since medical intervention, perhaps in the form of rehabilitation, is relevant to the relief of the impairment, whereas disability is usually understood within a social model, in which a disabling society imposes barriers or obstacles that prevent people with impairments from taking a full part in society. The medical model interprets impairment as a personal tragedy to be overcome by the individual through a combination of medical or technical assistance and personal courage, while the social model of disability looks to social reform to change the attitudes of society as a whole towards those who are regarded as disabled, thus leading to the removal of the obstructions, and the incorporation of impaired but no longer disabled people into the widest possible social life.[2] The medical

---

1 M. Bury, 'Defining and Researching Disability: Challenges and Responses', in C. Barnes and G. Mercer (eds), *Exploring the Divide: Illness and Disability*, Leeds: Disability Press, 1996, pp. 17–38, p. 19; C. Barnes, G. Mercer and T. Shakespeare, *Exploring Disability: A Sociological Introduction*, Cambridge: Polity Press, 1999, p. 27.

2 E. Morris and R. McCloughry, *Making a World of Difference: Christian Reflections on Disability*. London: SPCK, 2002, p. 14; M. Oliver, 'Defining

model leads to case history and autobiography whereas the social model leads to political action.³

A theology of impairment would be a branch of body theology,⁴ since it is the bodies and minds of people that are impaired. A theology of disability would be a branch of liberation theology since it would seek for social and political change for the emancipation of an oppressed group. The present study will argue that both kinds of theology are necessary, and that they are related. There would be a residual impact of impairment even if the objectives of social and political action by disabled people were completely successful. Even if British Sign Language (BSL) were more generally used in communication, and if the negative attitudes of society towards deafness were removed altogether, deaf people would still need light in order to interpret the gestures of those, whether hearing or deaf, who were in communication with them; and blind people would still lack the experience of colour even if freely provided with computerized synthetic speech. Advocates of the social model of disability have sometimes been nervous lest an emphasis upon the phenomenology of impairment might lead to a renewed interpretation of impairment in terms of personal tragedy for which nothing but courage and technology were necessary, and would distract attention away from the character of the disabling society.⁵ I hope to do something to minimize this fear by showing that a theological and philosophical awareness of impairment should lead to a wider understanding of the many forms taken by human life, and so to a more inclusive social policy for liberation.

There are two approaches to understanding the impaired body. The first is epistemological, dealing with the bodily basis of what we know, and the second is phenomenological, dealing with the nature of the subjectivity of impairment. The two approaches

Impairment and Disability: Issues at Stake', in C. Barnes and G. Mercer (eds), *Exploring the Divide: Illness and Disability*, Leeds: Disability Press, 1996, pp. 39–54, pp. 42–3.

3 Barnes, Mercer and Shakespeare, *Exploring Disability*, pp. 67ff.

4 J. B. Nelson, *Body Theology*, Louisville: Westminster/John Knox Press, 1992; L. Isherwood and E. Stuart, *Introducing Body Theology*, Sheffield: Sheffield Academic Press, 1998.

5 Oliver, 'Defining Impairment and Disability', p. 54.

converge in the work of the phenomenological epistemologist Maurice Merleau-Ponty.[6]

A Body Knows

Recent developments in brain research and cognitive science have emphasized the embodied character of the human mind, and that the influence of the body upon the mind is mainly at the preconscious or unconscious levels, forming the metaphors without which abstract thought would not be possible. 'Reason, even in its most abstract form, makes use of, rather than transcends, our animal nature.'[7] Reason does not transcend the body; it arises from it: body is expressed in mind. This is the reverse of the Hegelian idea that mind expresses itself in body, an idea that may be traced in the Christian tradition back at least as far as the Prologue of the Fourth Gospel. The human mind is not a computer because computers do not have bodies. This is their major disadvantage compared with humans. It is estimated that at least 95 per cent of the brain is continually occupied in the processing of millions of unconscious links.[8] Neural modelling, a concept within cognitive science, studies the neurological patterns that structure our bodily experience, making thought possible. Such fundamental concepts as back, front, up, down, around, in and out – all these and myriads of others are the building blocks of thought and are laid down by the experiences of our body in the world.[9] The truth is not merely that we need a body in order to think; it is that our very thoughts are the products of bodily processes.[10]

---

6 Maurice Merleau-Ponty, *Phenomenology of Perception*, London: Routledge and Kegan Paul, 1962; *The Primacy of Perception and Other Essays*, Evanston, IL: Northwestern University Press, 1964; *The Visible and the Invisible*, Evanston, IL: Northwestern University Press, 1968; H. Pietersma, *Phenomenological Epistemology*, Oxford: Oxford University Press, 2000.

7 G. Lakoff and M. Johnson, *Philosophy in the Flesh: The Embodied Mind and Its Challenge to Western Thought*, New York: Basic Books, 1999, p. 4.

8 Lakoff and Johnson, *Philosophy in the Flesh*, p. 13.

9 M. Johnson, *The Body in the Mind: The Bodily Basis of Meaning, Imagination and Reason*, London: University of Chicago Press, 1987.

10 Lakoff and Johnson, *Philosophy in the Flesh*, p. 37.

This approach to epistemology is saved from individual isolation by the fact that human beings share similar bodies, and can thus communicate meaningfully from body to body with or without spoken language. Thus our reasoning is capable of objectivity in the sense that it appeals to common human experience.[11] However, although similar, not all bodies are the same; indeed, no two bodies are exactly the same. Some bodies are male and others are female. Feminist writers have highlighted the way that men's experience is couched in a characteristic language, of which most men are unaware, since linguistic processing falls mostly within the 95 per cent of the brain that deals with such things. There are young bodies for whom the experience of being held by another or being thrown over father's shoulder, or having to squeeze between gigantic legs or encounter insuperable obstacles such as the rails around a cot, remain for ever imprinted upon the brain. Most significantly for our present purposes, there are blind bodies, deaf bodies, bodies with no legs or no arms, bodies with no feeling or movement below the neck, and bodies that survive only by means of medical appliances or medication. If all of our knowledge is embodied, the knowledge of those embodied in such different bodies must itself be different.

This leads to the proposition that those whose impairments are physical or sensory, to go no further afield, have knowledge of different human worlds. The person with schizophrenia lives in a different world, but this is not shared publicly, is not known by others as being their own world, and is regarded as a mental illness. The world as known by paraplegics, or deaf or blind people, is a world of objective knowledge because it is publicly known within these groups, and can be entered into through imagination and empathy by others. The world of blindness is distinctive but not mad. Moreover, the concept of 'world' implies a complex and integrated whole with many inhabitants. While it may be true in a weak sense that each of us inhabits his or her private world, the word can only be used in a strong sense

---

11 Johnson, *The Body in the Mind*, p. 175.

when there is something corporate and consistent about a point of view or an experience that is shared by many.

Let us examine the world that is constructed by the blind body and is shared by most of those who have this particular impairment.[12] It will be fuzzy around the edges because people are blind to various degrees, and become blind at various times in their lives. Speaking epistemologically, there is nothing a blind person knows that cannot also be known by a sighted person, but the reverse is not the case. Sighted people experience darkness but totally blind people do not experience light, nor can they. The experience of the blind knower, who lives in a world of tactile and aural stimuli, is concentrated upon touch and sound which, although in theory accessible by sighted people, is seldom experienced by them with such continuity and intensity. The blind knower has no colour, no perspective, no knowledge at a distance except when there is noise, no stars, no smiles, no microbes unless you get an infection, no mountains unless you climb one. We may thus describe the blind world as smaller than the sighted world, perhaps included within it because blind people cannot do or know anything that sighted people cannot, and yet possessing unique characteristics, like a well sunk in the sighted garden, or a black hole in the midst of a galaxy of brilliant stars.

The Life-World of Blind People

This leads us into the second strand of philosophical reflection, that which comes from phenomenology. Beginning with the subtle analyses of consciousness and intention of Edmund Husserl,[13] the study of the phenomena of memory, temporality and consciousness has led to the concept of the life-world. The phenomenological sociology created by Alfred Schütz[14]

---

12 W. P. Rowland, *Being Blind in the World: A Phenomenological Analysis of Blindness*, Pretoria: South African National Council for the Blind, 1985.

13 E. Husserl, *Cartesian Meditations: An Introduction to Phenomenology*, The Hague: Martinus Neihof, 1969.

14 A. Schütz, *The Phenomenology of the Social World*, Evanston, IL: Northwestern University Press, 1967; A. Schütz and T. Luckmann, *The Structures of the Life-World*, Evanston, IL: Northwestern University Press, 1973.

unravelled the way that such concepts as presence, contemporaneity and simultaneity may be used to unlock the characteristics of social relations, while the phenomenological psychiatry of Ludwig Binswanger concentrated upon mental illness as a dislocation of the fundamental experiences of space and time.[15] Thomas Luckmann described the life-world of religious people under the conditions of modernity.[16]

A rich literature of pathography has revealed the life-worlds of people with various impairments. These range from Oliver Sacks' detailed description of the experience of breaking a leg[17] to Melanie May's discovery of her identity as a lesbian Christian.[18] Central to these accounts is the experience of difference. Gay and lesbian people are not impaired but they may be disabled by a heterosexual society, which may be unable to accept such differences. The writings of Oliver Sacks,[19] remarkable for their detailed exploration of various neurological conditions, reveal a growing awareness of the fact that some differences, whether due to impairment or not, are so pronounced, stable and long-lasting that they may be described as distinct human worlds.

The worlds are themselves very different. The world of deaf people, for example, arises not so much out of an alleged impairment but from their being a linguistic minority, disabled by the negative and even hostile attitudes of the hearing world. As Jennifer Harris shows in her study of the deaf culture, there is a deaf construction of deafness which varies widely from the hearing construction of deafness, and the boundary between these two incompatible constructions is created by communication through signing.[20] Of course, if everybody in the society

---

15 L. Binswanger, *Being in the World: Selected Papers*, London: Souvenir Press, 1975.

16 T. Luckmann, *Life-world and Social Reality*, London: Heinemann Educational, 1983.

17 O. Sacks, *A Leg to Stand On*, London: Duckworth, 1984.

18 M. A. May, *A Body Knows: A Theo-poetics of Death and Resurrection*, New York: Continuum, 1995.

19 O. Sacks, *Seeing Voices: A Journey into the World of the Deaf*, Berkeley: University of California Press, 1973; *An Anthropologist on Mars*, London: Picador; 1989.

20 J. Harris, *The Cultural Meaning of Deafness*, Aldershot: Avebury, 1995, pp. 168ff.

used signing, the barrier would disappear and there would no longer be a contrast between an inside and an outside construction of deafness. The epistemic and life-world experiences of deaf people are no doubt more distinctive in societies where deafness functions as a linguistic minority than would be the case where deafness was completely accepted as natural in a society thoroughly permeated by signing. The experience of the deaf communities of Martha's Vineyard, an island off the coast of Massachusetts, suggests that, in spite of the fact that the knowledge deaf people have of the world is primarily visual, the ease of communication between themselves and their hearing companions tended to minimize this difference to the point where no one in the society was even conscious of it. In such a situation, deafness was not considered to be an impairment or a loss but merely a difference.[21] Many deaf people in Britain share this view, regarding deafness not so much as a loss of hearing but as a culture with its own language.

The world of blind people is not much like this. This is partly because there is no distinct blind language and therefore blind communities cannot be thought of as linguistic minorities. Braille is a code, not a language, and increasingly blind people read through the technology of synthetic speech and not so much through embossed scripts. Another reason why the blind world is less of a specific culture than the deaf world is that there is not so well developed a contrast between the blind construction of blindness and the sighted construction of blindness. There must be few blind people who would not agree that the loss of sight is a profound and impoverishing loss. The degree to which this makes the world of blindness distinctive is disputable. The sighted philosopher Brian Magee and the blind philosopher Martin Milligan exchanged a fascinating series of letters on this question, in which Milligan argued that the blind person's knowledge of the world is not imperfect compared with that of the sighted person, while Magee emphasized the different

---

21 Nora Ellen Groce, *Everyone Here Spoke Sign Language: Hereditary Deafness on Martha's Vineyard*, London: Harvard University Press, 1985.

cognitive conditions experienced by blind and sighted people.[22] The literature of blindness reveals a continuum from those who argue that blindness, like deafness, is a mere difference[23] to those like Magee and myself who argue that the difference is so significant that blindness may genuinely construct a different world.[24]

The Social and Political Implications of Impairment and Disability

The social and political significance of impairment when understood as a life-world with its own knowledge base lies in the demand to acknowledge difference, while the social and political significance of disability lies in the demand for justice and inclusion. The demand for an acknowledgement of difference is in partnership with the demand for inclusion, and the demand for inclusion must be satisfied without any diminution of difference, except that which is created by the unreformed disabling society. It is the denial of genuine difference that leads to exclusion. It is when the various worlds experienced by variously impaired people are not acknowledged but are regarded simply as deviations from the norm, or deficiencies to be understood in purely negative terms, that the exclusive tendencies of normality are at their most powerful. Activists in the various disabled communities are always struggling against the arrogance of the normal, the taken-for-granted canonicity of the average.

Sighted people seldom recognize the extent to which their world is the product of their visual bodies. 'The moment perception comes, my body effaces itself before it and never does perception grasp the body in the act of perceiving.'[25] Because

---

22 B. Magee and M. Milligan, *On Blindness: Letters Between Bryan Magee and Martin Milligan*, Oxford: Oxford University Press, 1995.

23 K. Jernigan, 'Blindness; Handicap or Characteristic?', *The Braille*, June 1974, pp. 289–97.

24 J. M. Hull, *On Sight and Insight: A Journey into the World of Blindness*, Oxford: One World, 1997; *In the Beginning There was Darkness: A Blind Person's Conversations with the Bible*, London: SCM Press, 2001; and Chapter 6 of the present volume.

25 Merleau-Ponty, *The Visible and the Invisible*, p. 9.

of this they can only regard non-visual persons as excluded to some extent from the human world by their tragic loss. While such an attitude persists, relations with blind people are likely to be patronizing and to show a suffocating surplus of compassion. If, however, one can distinguish between the experience of the loss of sight and the state of blindness, one can begin to realize the intrinsic character of the tactile and aural world, and to acknowledge that it is a legitimate human condition. Consider, for example, the implications for the distinctiveness of the blind condition of the fact that there is no recorded example of schizophrenia in the case of someone born blind.[26] To be deprived of sight is not to be deprived of soul.

A Christian Theology of the Impaired Body

Remembering the two strands of analysis with which we began, we must distinguish between the theological implications of the knowledge that the blind body has of itself and the world and, on the other hand, the phenomenology of the impaired body in its life-world. Let us begin by considering the impaired body in its special knowledge as a theological category. One of the South American liberation theologians has said that, although the poor as such are no nearer God than the rich, and have no deeper spirituality, they do possess a cognitive advantage: the poor know a world that is unknown to the rich; they know the truth about society in a manner that is concealed from the wealthy. The poor are not particularly blessed for having that knowledge; indeed, no one actually desires such knowledge, and it may lead to bitterness or violence, but at least they are closer to the truth than are the rich. That proximity to truth is the starting point for what Paulo Freire called the ontological vocation of human beings,[27] and it was at that point that he began his famous pedagogy of the oppressed.

---

26 A. Stevens and J. Price, *Evolutionary Psychiatry: A New Beginning*, second edition, London: Routledge, 2000, p. 232.
27 P. Freire, *Pedagogy of the Oppressed*, London: Sheed and Ward, 1972, p. 21.

Impaired people have a similar advantage. First, they know that there is a plurality of human worlds. This knowledge is largely hidden from the multitude. Since the path to human solidarity lies through the recognition of human plurality, the knowledge that impaired people have is a vital clue to the humanizing of the future.

Second, the impaired body knows the meaning of difference and otherness in a world where the assumption of sameness is allied to the insensitivity of the powerful.

Third, the impaired body knows smallness, limitation, ignorance, and possibly pain. Indeed, such knowledge is itself painful, and does not in itself bring blessing to impaired people. This knowledge, like the other knowledge that the impaired body has of the world and of itself, may lead to isolation and bitterness, but if this can be overcome the knowledge may lead to precious insights and new impulses for reform. 'Only power that springs from the weakness of the oppressed will be sufficiently strong to free both.'[28]

The Christian faith can offer only limited support to such impaired body-knowledge. Just as the Christian faith finds itself on both sides of the struggle between the rich and the poor, so it finds itself on both sides of the knowledge of the impaired body and that of the non-impaired body.[29] So much of the Bible presents us with non-impaired body-knowledge: human beings are created with perfect bodies, sin enters the world and with it impairment, Jesus as the apocalyptic redeemer restores impaired bodies, and impairment will be banished in the world to come.

On the other hand, the central symbol of the Christian faith is a broken body, remembered in the broken bread and the poured-out wine.[30] The deeper mysteries of the Christian faith are ill at odds with the mythology of a perfection lost and regained, for the resurrected, ascended and glorified body is still wounded and still imperfect. Our human impaired bodies represent our broken humanity in the presence of a vulnerable God. Before

---

28 Freire, *Pedagogy of the Oppressed*, p. 28.
29 See Chapter 6 and Chapter 8 of the present volume.
30 See Chapter 6 (above).

the throne there stands a lamb as if slain (Rev. 5.6, 12). This strange vision of vulnerability lies at the heart of the message to the weakened Saint Paul, to whom the Lord said, 'My grace is sufficient for you, for power is made perfect in weakness' (2 Cor. 12.9). In other words, the ability of God is made perfect through disability.

A Theological Approach to the Phenomenology of the Impaired Life-World

A theology of the life-worlds of impaired people transforms the epistemological insights into the rounded reality of daily human experience. Of course, no human being is totally enclosed within a single life-world, but each possesses many finite provinces of meaning.[31] We live in the everyday world, and also in the world of dreams, the world of theatre and film, and the world of religious experience. Blindness is only one aspect of a blind person's life. A blind person is certainly an impaired motorist but not an impaired telephone user. A person who is blind may also be active in politics or in business. The life-world of a blind person is intersected by other life-worlds in which the same person lives; or, to put it in a different way, we have many identities, and each identity has its own narrative.

The plurality of the life-worlds is reflected in the creative work of God who made the earth abound with many forms of life (Gen. 1.20–25), who knows and respects the mysterious, wild forms of life, and calls each to be faithful to its own nature (Job 38.39—39.30). The life-worlds are reflected in the diversity of the callings of various ministries in the Church, where each life-world is a gift, and each gift is a vocation (1 Cor. 12.4–11). The life-worlds of the men and women around him were respected by Jesus, the founder of the community of inclusive love.[32] He saw Nathanael when he was in his private world (John 1.47f.),

---

31 Schütz and Luckmann, *Structures of the Life-world*, pp. 21ff.

32 G. Theissen, *A Theory of Primitive Christian Religion*, London: SCM Press, 1999, pp. 64–71.

he understood the life-history of the woman he met at the well (John 4.17–18), and he called people from the worlds they knew into new worlds (Mark 1.19–20), to a new creation (2 Cor. 5.17).

A Theology Against a Disabling Society

We have been discussing some of the ways that lead from a theology of impairment to a theology of disability. Theology of impairment represents a demand for a recognition of otherness, and for a solidarity that includes without denying difference. This is a protest against the disabling society which insists upon the power of the many, which in the end becomes the power of the few. In the struggle for this social and political renewal, the Christian faith offers the model of the Holy Trinity, as a society of different but equal persons in the single unity of the one God. Difference is recognized, for the Father is not the Son, and the Son is not the Spirit; and the different callings are emphasized, for the Father is the ground of all being, and the Son is made flesh and is broken, while the Holy Spirit is the Lord, the giver of life. Yet all are incorporated into a single, blissful unity of which the circular dance is the symbol, as expressed by the early Church theologians with the Greek word *perichoresis*.

In addition, in seeking equality and social justice for disabled people, the Christian faith offers a whole range of images and concepts, which may often have little specific reference to disability but are nevertheless a resource for the religiously motivated social activist.

What Difference Does It Make?

Can such a theology make a difference? Yes, and this may happen in two ways. First, in so far as the Christian faith, in many of its received forms, is part of the problem, and is often an unconscious collaborator with the disabling society, we can speak of a disabling faith. When persons of faith become disabled, this disabling faith is internalized and often becomes conscious, adding to the loss of identity and self-esteem. If Christian theology can become more inclusive, impaired people within this tradition will be liberated to a certain extent.

Second, the influence of the Christian churches throughout the world is still considerable. If the energies of this great international movement can be revitalized and directed in a more coherent way against the disabling society, disabled activists will have found a powerful ally and, from the Christian point of view, a step will have been taken towards the realization of the Kingdom of God.

8

The Broken Body in a Broken World

A Contribution to a Christian Doctrine of the Person from a Disabled Point of View

Finding a Starting Point: Image or Body?

From a disabled point of view, there are difficulties in using the concept of the image of God as a starting point for a Christian understanding of the person. These difficulties have to do with the perfection that is suggested by the analogy. The image of God as portrayed in the Bible is that of a being whose perfect knowledge is attained through the perfection of the divine senses. When Hezekiah prays, 'Incline your ear, O LORD, and hear; open your eyes, O LORD, and see' (Isa. 37.17), the assumption is not that God is hard of hearing or has a sight defect. God never has a mobility problem. 'If I ascend to heaven, you are there; if I make my bed in Sheol, you are there' (Ps. 139.8). It is generally recognized today that locating the image of God mainly in the intellect is unsatisfactory because it limits the degree to which slow learners and people with mental disorders can be thought of as being in God's image. However, even when the image of God is conceived of as residing in such human attributes as the capacity to love or to possess imagination and freedom, there is a tendency to create a kind of sliding scale such that those whose freedom is impaired by disability and those whose capacity to love is impaired by pain are more or less excluded. If the image of God is conceived of as residing in relationality, then those whose human relations are damaged are at a disadvantage. Of course, it is agreed that the image of God has been defaced by sin, but the problem is that, because of a persistent tendency to infer inner sinful states from outer imperfections, disabled people tend to be regarded as particular evidences of the fall of Adam and Eve. This is why the eschatological vision describes the removal of disabilities. 'Then the eyes of the blind shall be opened, and the ears of the deaf unstopped; then the lame shall leap like a deer, and the tongue of the speechless sing for joy' (Isa. 35.5–6). Because God is perfect, the image of God must be found in that which is perfect, or in that which is moving towards perfection. The problem lies in the fact that the divine perfection is imaged upon, or is a projection of, the ideals of a perfect human being or a perfect human life. It is this convergent or unequivocal model of perfection, this implicit refusal to acknowledge the multiplicity of the genuinely human, that leads many disabled people to search for a different starting point for a Christian theology of the person.[1]

From Image to Body

The main purpose of the present study is to suggest that the real humanity of disabled people might be better protected if we take as our starting point not the image of God but the human body itself. That is not to deny that the idea that all human life is sacred because 'made in the image of God' is a significant defence against all attempts to diminish the humanity of any human being. Nevertheless, if we were to complement a theology of the human drawn from the *imago Dei* with an anthropology drawn from the human body certain advantages would follow.

However, an immediate disadvantage springs to mind. The *imago Dei* safeguards the uniqueness of human beings by indicating such human characteristics as the capacity for freedom and love, or the human responsibility as the steward of creation, whereas the human body is similar to the bodies of other species. In this sense, starting a Christian doctrine of the person from the image of God seems to protect the distinctively human,

---

[1] I have explored the implications of the idea of the perfect human face and having visual access to the face in Chapter 5 of the present volume.

but starting from the body seems to lose the human in a more general biological category.

On the other hand, perhaps this is not a bad thing. When we speak disparagingly of our animal nature, we insult animals. Our animal nature refers, so we think, to our capacity for cruelty, murder and lust; but animals have needs not lusts, kill only to eat, and are incapable of deliberately planned cruelty. Moreover, to start our thinking from the body enables our theology to develop intimately with the study of biology, and recent work in the biological origins of religion makes this an attractive option.[2] Finally, when we begin our theological anthropology from the body, we are drawn immediately into such central Christian symbols as the body of Christ, which links anthropology not only to the incarnation but also to the Church and the sacraments. A Christian theological anthropology based upon the body thus has a number of advantages.

Body Theology as a Theology of Disability

Although a distinction is sometimes made[3] between physical disability, meaning for example the loss of limbs or the loss of bodily functions, and (on the other hand) sensory disability (loss of sight or hearing) and mental disability including mental illness and psychological disorder, there is an important sense in which all disability is physical. It is the body that is disabled, whether one thinks of the brain, the eye or the foot as being a disabled organ. A characteristic of the experience of disability is that one becomes particularly sensitive to one's body. My twenty-one-year-old son told me that he never really noticed that he had legs until he broke one of his feet in a fall and had to use crutches for three months. Of course, the embodied character of disability is not its only feature, and many disabled people claim that it is the social rather than the physical aspects of disability that are most

---

[2] Anthony Stevens and John Price, *Evolutionary Psychiatry: A New Beginning*, London: Routledge, 2000.

[3] *World Programme of Action Concerning Disabled Persons* [U. N. Decade of Disabled Persons 1982–1992], New York: United Nations, 1983, I.c. 6–7.

alienating. My son not only discovered his legs; he discovered that he could not carry a pint of beer from the bar to the table where his friends were seated, and was left feeling foolish standing by the bar wondering if someone would come and help him.

One must also realize that the degree to which a physical condition is disabling is affected by the surrounding culture. A woman who could not walk more than half a mile would be considered normal in, say, Los Angeles, where her limitation would not be noticed, but in a village community, perhaps in parts of Africa, where women were expected to walk several miles each day fetching water for their families, someone who could walk only half a mile would be severely disabled.[4] The study of disability is therefore an inter-disciplinary enquiry, involving not only physiology and psychology but also sociology and cultural studies. Nevertheless these various disciplines all involve an interpretation of the body under certain conditions. Whatever the discipline, disability studies involve hermeneutics, and the text of disabled hermeneutics is the body.

The Body as Epistemic Reality

The body is a suitable starting point for a Christian anthropology and especially for a theology of disability, not only because disability sits, as it were, in the body, but because the body is the source of our knowledge not only of ourselves but of the world and everything in it. In other words, the body is an epistemic principle. An older epistemology regarded human knowledge as founded in absolute ideas or transcendental realities, whether those of Plato or of Hegel, which were merely received by human beings. The British empirical epistemology regarded human knowledge as coming to us through our bodily senses, but it did not emphasize or understand the contribution that our own bodies make to the character and reception of this sense-based knowledge. Much twentieth-century linguistic philosophy

---

4 Susan Wendall, *The Rejected Body: Feminist Philosophical Reflections on Disability*, London: Routledge, 1996, p. 14.

regarded knowledge as being expressed in propositions. Knowledge always takes a linguistic form. Truth abides in words. Only sentences can express truthful ideas. While it is possible that all three theories of knowledge do make a contribution to understanding the character of human knowledge, more recent philosophical work has drawn attention to the body itself as the locus and origin of knowledge.[5] This emphasis upon the body is a development of the constructivist epistemology, in which human knowledge is regarded as a human creation. Human knowledge is created by humans. Human knowledge takes the form of constructs, which express the social and political position of the knower. The emphasis upon bodily knowledge takes this further by pointing out that we know the world as our bodies know it.[6]

This is important for a philosophy and a theology of disability because it enables us to postulate the existence of several worlds of human knowledge. The experience that a blind person has of the world is so significantly different from that of sighted people that we can speak of it as a constructed world. This emphasizes the independence and integrity, the wholeness of the blind world, and sets blindness free from being interpreted merely in terms of deficiency. Blindness is not just something that happens to one's eyes; it is something that happens to one's world. This enables us also to relativize the hegemonic assumptions of many sighted people, who do not always realize that they live in a world that is a projection of their sighted bodies, but make the mistake of thinking that the world is just like that, the way they see it. Such people are never able to respect or understand blind people, but will always regard them as being merely excluded from the sighted world, and not as having a more or less independent world of their own.[7]

---

5 Mark Johnson, *The Body in the Mind: The Bodily Basis of Meaning, Imagination, and Reason*, London: University of Chicago Press, 1987, and Mark Johnson and George Lakoff (eds), *Philosophy in the Flesh: The Embodied Mind and Its Challenge to Western Thought*, New York: Basic Books, 1999.

6 Maurice Merleau-Ponty, *Phenomenology of Perception*, London: Routledge and Kegan Paul, 1962.

7 I have explored the idea of blindness as being a more or less distinct world of human experience elsewhere in this book, in Chapters 4, 5, and especially Chapter 6.

The significance of this for Christian anthropology lies in the fact that it emphasizes the plurality of human worlds, and the recognition of the plurality immediately relativizes the absolute claims of a single, dominant world. There are many kinds of human bodies, some young, some old, some male, others female, some with arms and legs, others without arms or legs, some who hear, others who do not hear, some who are rich and others who are poor, some who oppress others and some who are oppressed. This enables us to make a further distinction between the human worlds that are, so to speak, natural in that they spring from the body as natural body-knowledge, and (on the other hand) those worlds that have no bodily basis, no natural epistemological character, but are the social constructions of power and greed. When we recognize natural epistemic worlds, we can also recognize unnatural ones. It is true that the rich and poor know different worlds, but this is an epistemic distinction stemming from the experience of injustice; it is also true that the blind and the sighted know different worlds, but this is a natural epistemic distinction, stemming from the physical characteristics of the blind and sighted body. The distinctive character of the blind world may be further emphasized by the fact that many blind people are economically disadvantaged. Blind people who live in poverty live in a world of blindness that is shared by wealthy blind people, but they also live in a socially generated world of poverty. The unnaturally generated economic worlds should be criticized and rejected but the bodily worlds of blindness and deafness should be understood and respected.

We see then that a Christian anthropology must begin by emphasizing the relativizing impact of plurality. Only when this is done can the experiences of disabled people be honoured as making a positive contribution to the fullness of human life, and only when this is done can the artificial divisions between unnatural human worlds be recognized for what they are – the disembodied shadows of evil which settle upon and oppress human bodies. The affirmation of one category of world makes possible the denunciation of another category.

This is one of the reflections that have led to the appearance of body theology as a genre of theological literature.[8] Of course, not all body theology springs from the epistemology I have described. Much of it is motivated by a rejection of the older Christian tradition that tended to dismiss the body, regarding it as the source of evil temptation and sin. Body theology is often an attempt to reclaim the wholeness of the human person.[9] Much body theology comes from women's theology, and challenges the domination of male ways of understanding the world. By emphasizing the characteristics of the female body, the female theologians have drawn attention to the characteristics of the female life cycle, the female experience of life and women's religious experience.[10] Other contributions of body theology are motivated by a desire to re-interpret Christian ethics in a more realistic sense, emphasizing the homophobic character of much traditional Christian sexual ethics.[11] Body theology also regards itself as a theology of the incarnation, emphasizing the embodied character of the divine revelation in which the word became flesh.

While not all theologies of disability can be regarded as examples of body theology,[12] there is no doubt that many of the most powerful interpretations of disability express epistemological aspects of body experience.[13] They may not be specifically theo-

---

8 Although certainly not a theological author, Nancy Hartsock should be mentioned as her work is of considerable significance in understanding capitalist and feminist epistemologies as springing from relationships of power in society. Nancy C. M. Hartsock, *Money, Sex and Power: Toward a Feminist Historical Materialism*, London: Longman, 1983, pp. 231ff. and *passim*.

9 James B. Nelson, *Body Theology*, Louisville, KY: Westminster/John Knox Press, 1992.

10 Lisa Isherwood and Elizabeth Stuart, *Introducing Body Theology*, Sheffield: Sheffield Academic Press, 1998.

11 James B. Nelson, *Embodiment: An Approach to Sexuality and Christian Theology*, London: SPCK, 1979.

12 For example, David Pailin offers a theology of disability based upon process philosophy. David A. Pailin, *A Gentle Touch: From a Theology of Handicap to a Theology of Human Being*, London: SPCK, 1992.

13 For example, Barbara B. Patterson, 'Redeemed Bodies, Fullness of Life', in Nancy L. Eiesland and Don E. Saliers (eds), *Human Disability and the Service of God: Reassessing Religious Practice*, Nashville: Abingdon Press, 1998, pp. 123ff. is mainly concerned with the nature of Christ's resurrected body. Some contributions to theology of disability emphasize the character and consequences of exclusion: Don E. Saliers, 'Toward a Spirituality of Inclusiveness' and Jürgen Moltmann,

logical but spring from twentieth-century philosophical schools such as phenomenology and existentialism. This is why in our search for a Christian anthropology we must go beyond a philosophy of the disabled body and find a specifically Christian theology.

Why Is a Theology of Disability Necessary?

The search for a theology of disability arises from the fact that Christian disabled people, often inspired by contemporary social and philosophical approaches towards an understanding of disability, are dissatisfied with the place that disability occupies in many interpretations of the Christian faith. The miracles of Jesus in healing disabled people are not always regarded by disabled people as offering them hope[14] but on the contrary are looked upon as encouraging an attitude of charity and of mission towards them. Many disabled people feel that their human dignity is taken from them by the expectation that they should, as Christians, be healed by Christ. This brings us to the connection between disability and sin. In spite of frequent denials, disabled people in many cultures report that they are often regarded as deficient in faith, or as having positively sinned.[15]

The connection between disability and sin goes much deeper than the suspicion that with a little bit more faith disabled people could be miraculously restored. It is rooted in the biblical view of the world, which became the basis for an articulate structure of Christian doctrine. This describes a cosmic history falling into three distinct periods. In the first period, the created universe was in a state of blissful perfection. Adam and Eve in

---

'Liberate Yourselves by Accepting One Another' in the same volume. Others derive inspiration from theology of liberation: Nancy L. Eiesland, *The Disabled God: Toward a Liberatory Theology of Disability*, Nashville: Abingdon Press, 1994.

14 John M. Hull, *In the Beginning There Was Darkness: A Blind Person's Conversations with the Bible*, London: SCM Press, 2001 and Harrisburg, PA: Trinity Press International, 2002.

15 Anecdotes from several countries were reported by members of the Ecumenical Disability Advocates Network of the World Council of Churches meeting in Cartigny, Switzerland, 1-5 October 2001.

the Garden of Eden were in a state of perfect humanity, unblemished in their bodies, in their relationships with each other and in their communion with God. The second period runs from the fall of Adam and Eve through to the second coming of Christ and the Day of Judgement. The Bible is almost wholly concerned with this second period, which is the story of redemption. It is the period of grace, including the election of Israel and the calling into existence of the Church after the death and resurrection of Jesus Christ. The third and final period will be the consummation of history, when once again pain and evil will be banished and human beings will again be in perfect communion with God in a restored creation, much more enduring than the first condition since the human state will be transformed by the vision of God.[16]

In this scheme of things, there is no place for disabled people in either the first or the final worlds. Disability is a characteristic of the second age. Although disabled people may not necessarily have sinned or brought their condition upon themselves through their own sin or that of their parents, their very existence is a continual reminder of the imperfect human condition, into which humanity has fallen and from which we hope to be redeemed. Even when the connection is not with sin itself, disability is associated with an imperfect world, a sort of natural disaster like earthquakes and hunger and death itself, indicative of a disturbed creation. Hence the expectation that in the Messianic age the lame will leap like a hart and the tongues of the dumb shall sing (Isa. 35.5–6). Everything will be restored as creation, which at present groans in its bondage, is brought into the full liberty of the sons and daughters of God (Rom. 8.19).

It is this belief, often expressed through a more-or-less unconscious attitude towards disability itself, that becomes attached to disabled people. Men and women, boys and girls with disabilities become the concrete instances of a general phenomenon of disability which itself is part of the imperfect world. It is because

---

16 This view of the Christian myth was a characteristic of the federal theology which by 1600 had become the main type of Reformed theology in Western Europe. David A. Weir, *The Origins of the Federal Theology in Sixteenth Century Reformation Thought*, Oxford: Clarendon Press, 1990, especially pp. 62ff.

of associations such as these that many disabled people have come to believe that, far from being a power for their emancipation, the Christian faith is a major source of the social and economic disadvantage that they suffer. The Christian faith, to put it more bluntly, is seen not as part of the answer but as part of the problem. This is why disabled people who wish to regard themselves as disciples of Jesus Christ and to remain within the Christian Church are struggling to formulate various theologies of disability.

Resources for a Theology of Disability

While it is true that Christian theology has elements that appear to exclude and marginalize people with disabilities, the situation is far from simple. The Christian faith is a complex web of texts, traditions and symbols which to some extent defies systematization, as is indicated by the thousands of Christian denominations. There are even theologians who regard the very concept of a systematic theology as being un-Christian. Moreover, the constant re-interpretation of aspects of the Christian faith, a process without which it would no longer be a living stream of human experience and a continuing revelation, means that some aspects of faith become disjointed from others. It is the constant task of systematics to restore and reunify faith. The result of this is that the Christian faith has become for us a huge resource of ideas, lives and traditions, from which the modern believer, whether a woman, or a black person, or a person suffering oppression, or a disabled person, can pick and mix. Peter Berger has described this situation as a heretical imperative,[17] and Robert Bellah has distinguished between the compact symbolism of earlier Christian periods and the complex symbolism of our own.[18]

---

17 Peter L. Berger, *The Heretical Imperative: Contemporary Possibilities of Religious Affirmation*, London: Collins, 1980.
18 Robert N. Bellah, *Beyond Belief: Essays on Religion in a Post-Traditional World*, London: Harper & Row, 1970, Chapter 2, 'Religious Evolution'.

So it is that the Christian person with a disability in search of a theology may find that, although the symbols of the fall, the miraculous healings and the Eschaton are not helpful, there are other symbols which may offer more constructive suggestions. For example, the apostle Paul is much maligned for his negative attitudes towards the ministry of women but is to be praised for his interpretations of disability. It may be that Paul himself had a disability, or had experienced some painful loss, possibly a partial loss of sight.[19] There is no doubt that Paul was extremely conscious of the body. There is no other biblical author who speaks so frequently and with such a variety of images of the body as does Paul.[20]

The Body in Pauline Thought

Paul shows a striking sensitivity towards the body. For example, sexual malpractice (as Paul understood it) is not simply unethical but dishonours the bodies of those who engage in it (Rom. 1.24). The body of an old man is practically dead because the man is no longer capable of procreation (Rom. 4.19), but if a man has intercourse with a prostitute he becomes one body with her (1 Cor. 6.16). Once again, it is not exactly the moral consideration, or the possibly harmful effect of such a relationship upon the parties, but the way it creates a rather unpleasant body for the one who has relations with the prostitute. 'Every sin that a person commits is outside the body; but the fornicator sins against the body itself' (1 Cor. 6.18). It is in the body that sin reigns (Rom. 6.12) and therefore it can be called a 'body of sin' (Rom. 6.6), and thus 'the body is dead because of sin' (Rom. 8.10). It is a 'lowly body' or 'a body of humiliation' (Phil. 3.21).

The Christian faith redeems the body (Rom. 8.23); the body belongs to the Lord and the Lord to the body (1 Cor. 6.13). The body of a Christian has become the temple of the Holy Spirit

---

19 Hull, *In The Beginning*, pp. 52–8.
20 I am grateful to Professor Troels Engberg-Pedersen of the University of Copenhagen for sending me a copy of his paper 'Body Language in Paul', which he presented to the British New Testament Conference in Manchester on 6–8 September 2001.

(1 Cor. 6.19) and consequently Christians are to glorify God in their bodies (1 Cor. 6.20).

Paul imagines that his body has the functions of a woman's body (Gal. 4.19). And he hopes that Christ will be exalted in his body, whether in life or death (Phil. 1.20). When the Spirit or breath enters into the bodies of Christians, they are given life in spite of their mortality (Rom. 8.11). It is the body of the believer that is to be presented to God as a living sacrifice (Rom. 12.1).

These passages indicate the curious emphasis that Paul places upon the body, often speaking of the body when we today would more naturally refer to our lives, rather than our bodies. It is possible that this sensitivity was produced by Paul's own experience of physical suffering, loss or disability. He carries the marks of Jesus branded on his body (Gal. 6.17), and he is conscious of always carrying in his body the death of Jesus, so that the life of Jesus might be made visible in his body (2 Cor. 4.10). Of course, such expressions may refer to the persecutions which the Christian missionaries suffered – Paul often uses the plural. There is no doubt, however, about the personal nature of the experience reported in 2 Corinthians 12.7, the thorn in the flesh. These expressions may refer to the scars or wounds caused by the Roman beatings or possibly to some other type of physical infirmity. We can be sure of this: all experiences of these kinds tend to make us acutely conscious of our bodies.

When we consider the number of references to the body in Paul's letters (and we have referred only to a few of them), it becomes possible to consider the theology of Paul as an example of body theology. Paul's theological epistemology appears to have been grounded in his body, in life as his body knew it.

The Broken Body of Christ

It is this body theology that helps us to understand the intense attraction that Paul felt for the body of Jesus Christ. Just as he knew the world that his own body knew, he was grasped by the world that the body of Jesus knew. His body, indeed, had become the body of Jesus, bearing upon it the marks that the body of Jesus bore. Jesus had delivered him from his body of death (Rom. 7.24) and one day his body of humiliation would become like the glorified body of Christ (Phil. 3.21). His physical body would become a spiritual body (1 Cor. 15.44). The body of Christ was to be found as the Church (1 Cor. 12.27), since baptism had joined all believers into one body (1 Cor. 12.13). So vivid was Paul's sense of Christians having actually become the body of Christ that the concept became an argument against prostitution, not as a matter of obedience to a commandment or consistency with a life of discipleship, but because it would be impossible to take members of Christ and make them members of a prostitute (1 Cor. 6.15).

The central feature of Paul's body-knowledge of Jesus' body-knowledge was that it was broken. '[W]hen he had given thanks, he broke it and said, "This is my body that is for you. Do this in remembrance of me"' (1 Cor. 11.24). This is the earliest record of what took place at the Last Supper, and brokenness lies at the heart of it. It is because of its brokenness that partakers of the bread proclaim the death of Christ (1 Cor. 11.26), for in his death he was broken. Not to discern the brokenness is not to discern the body of Christ (1 Cor. 11.29). It is because the original unity is broken into a multiplicity that the multiplicity becomes a unity. 'Because there is one bread, we who are many are one body, for we all partake of the one bread' (1 Cor. 10.17). The unity of the Church is recreated again and again as the broken body is restored into the oneness of Christ's body the Church.

It is not only in the emphatic body theology of Paul that we find this meaning of brokenness. In all three synoptic Gospels Jesus is described as breaking the bread at the Last Supper (Matt. 26.26; Mark 14.22; Luke 22.19). The story of the feeding of the crowd with the loaves and fishes evidently made a great impression upon the early Church since variations of it are recorded no fewer than five times in the synoptic Gospels, and in every case the breaking of the bread is referred to (Matt. 14.19, 15.36; Mark 6.41, 8.6; Luke 9.13). The eucharistic significance of the miracle is made clear through the repetition of the sequence of prayer, breaking and distributing in both the miracle and in all three synoptic accounts of the Last Supper.

THE BROKEN BODY IN A BROKEN WORLD

The significance of the brokenness for understanding the meaning of the death of Jesus is reinforced in Mark by the story of the woman who broke an alabaster jar of very costly ointment and poured it upon the head of Jesus (Mark 14.3). The breaking of the jar is unique to Mark, who links the event with the burial of the body of Jesus (Mark 14.8). This may be an example of Pauline influence upon the Gospel of Mark, where as we have seen the brokenness of the body of Jesus is a prominent theme. It may be significant that neither Matthew nor Luke says that the jar of ointment was broken (Matt. 26.7; Luke 7.38), and Luke, who brings the story further forward in his Gospel, does not connect it with the burial at all. It was necessary to break the jar in order to release the fragrance of the ointment, and it was necessary to break the body in order to release the life of Jesus for the world.

Although Luke has his own interpretation of the incident in which the woman anoints Jesus with perfume, he is fully aware of the significance of the breaking of the bread as a moment of revelation in which the presence of the crucified and risen Jesus is realized. It is when the unrecognized companion breaks the bread that the disciples know him (Luke 24.30–31). Once again, the ritual sequence of blessing, breaking and distributing is referred to. The two disciples do not report to the others that Jesus had appeared to them on the road or that he had spoken with them, but only that 'he had been made known to them in the breaking of the bread' (Luke 24.35). More than once in Luke's account of the early Church, we are told of the breaking of bread. This was done with gladness of heart at home or from house to house (Acts 2.46); it became a regular feature of the Sunday evening meeting of the church (Acts 20.7); and, in the presence of the terrified sailors during the storm, Paul 'took bread; and giving thanks to God in the presence of all, he broke it and began to eat' (Acts 27.35) as an indication of his confidence in their escape.

The interpretation of brokenness is quite different in John, where it is specifically stated that the legs of Jesus were not broken (John 19.31–33). Indeed, John regards this as a fulfilment of Psalm 34.20, 'None of his bones shall be broken' (John

19.36). Moreover, the Fourth Gospel not only makes no reference to the breaking of the bread at the Last Supper, but does not mention the bread and the wine at all. The Johannine account of the miraculous feeding does not refer to the breaking of the bread (John 6.11). We have the usual blessing, followed by the distribution, but no breaking. John's account is modelled upon the manna that came down from heaven. It was given, but not broken (John 6.48–51). When we turn to the story of the woman with the jar of ointment, we find that not only is the jar not broken, it is not even mentioned (John 12.2–8). In view of the significance that Luke attaches to the breaking of the bread, we should almost certainly regard his failure to say that the jar was broken as insignificant. After all, Luke says that there was a jar and, since the woman anoints Jesus, the jar or the seal must have been broken. By way of contrast, John avoids this implication by making the jar disappear. He speaks simply of 'a pound of costly perfume' (John 12.3). Little details add up, and if we want to get a full picture of John's Gospel on this point we must turn from the concept of brokenness to that of wounding. Only the Fourth Gospel tells us that Jesus was wounded in the side (John 19.34). John is quite emphatic about this. 'He who saw this has testified so you also may believe. His testimony is true' (John 19.35), and it is possible that the ambiguous words that follow call upon God to witness to its truth.

'Rich Wounds Yet Visible Above'

The hymn 'Crown him with many crowns' by Matthew Bridges (1800–94) is a meditation upon Christ the King. The exaltation of the ascended Christ is referred to in the Nicene Creed with the words, 'He ascended into heaven, and is seated at the right hand of the Father. He will come again in glory to judge the living and the dead, and his kingdom will have no end.' The third verse of the hymn is:

> Crown him the Lord of love;
> Behold his hands and side,

> Those wounds yet visible above
> In beauty glorified:
> No angel in the sky
> Can fully bear that sight,
> But downward bends his burning eye
> At mysteries so bright.

A later verse concludes:

> His reign shall know no end,
> And round his pierced feet
> Fair flowers of Paradise extend
> Their fragrance ever sweet.[21]

In the previous century, Charles Wesley (1707–88) wrote 'Lo, he comes with clouds descending'. One verse reads:

> Those dear tokens of his passion
> Still his dazzling body bears,
> Cause of endless exultation
> To his ransomed worshippers:
> With what rapture
> Gaze we on those glorious scars!

One of the bases of the doctrine of the wounded heavenly body of Christ is Zechariah 12.10: 'when they look on the one whom they have pierced, they shall mourn for him'. It is this text that Wesley refers to in a previous verse of the famous Advent hymn.

> Every eye shall now behold him,
> Robed in dreadful majesty;
> Those who set at naught and sold him,
> Pierced and nailed him to the tree,
> Deeply wailing
> Shall the true Messiah see.[22]

---

21 *Common Praise*, Norwich: Canterbury Press, 2000, no. 166.
22 *Common Praise*, no. 31.

The source of this doctrine is to be found in the Gospels of Luke and John. Both tell us that the scars or wounds of Jesus were still visible in his resurrected body. In Luke we read that Jesus said to the fearful disciples:

> 'Look at my hands and feet; see that it is I myself. Touch me and see; for a ghost does not have flesh and bones as you see that I have.' And when he had said this, he showed them his hands and his feet. (Luke 24.39–40)

No doubt the scarred hands and feet were prominent among the 'many convincing proofs' by means of which 'he presented himself alive to them' (Acts 1.3). The question is whether, if the scars were visible in the resurrected body, they were also visible in the ascended body. This question, strange as it is to most modern people, presented a gift to the devout imagination of earlier generations of Christians.[23] After all, did not the angels say, 'This Jesus, who has been taken up from you into heaven, will come in the same way as you saw him go into heaven' (Acts 1.11)? The King James Bible translates it 'This same Jesus ...', which leads to the thought that the identity of the returning Christ will be verifiable by the same scars, now glorious as Wesley said, and beautiful as Bridges says. This is the basis of the belief that those who pierced him will behold with horror the scars that witness to their cruelty.

The idea of the wounded resurrected body is even more vivid in the Fourth Gospel. As we have seen, only John refers to Jesus being wounded in the side, and Bridges' hymn says, 'behold his hands and side'. Only in John does Thomas demand proof of the identity of the resurrected man with the crucified man by asking to see his wounds. 'Unless I see the mark of the nails in his hands, and put my finger in the mark of the nails and my hand in his side, I will not believe' (John 20.25). When the resurrected Jesus appears a week later he says to Thomas 'Put your finger here and see my hands. Reach out your hand and put it in my side. Do not doubt but believe' (John 20.27). The astonishing

---

23 The doctrine of the scarred resurrected body in the early Christian centuries is discussed by Barbara Patterson, 'Redeemed Bodies', p. 126.

thing about these words is that they presuppose a deep wound in the side of Jesus. To put one's finger on and to see the hands is consistent with scarring, but to put one's hand into the wound suggests a wound that was still open. This is why the hymn does not speak of scars but of 'rich wounds, yet visible above'. We may wonder why God who had the power to raise the body of Jesus from the dead did not exercise the power to perfectly heal the body, but that is not the point. The continued visibility of the wounds was necessary in order to establish the identity of the person. True, Paul says that the body is 'perishable, what is raised is imperishable. It is sown in dishonour, it is raised in glory. It is sown in weakness, it is raised in power. It is sown a physical body, it is raised a spiritual body' (1 Cor. 15.42–44), but if we are to combine Paul with Luke and John we must add that the body of Christ is raised with imperishable scars, glorious scars, and in a state of wounded power. So we see that this biblical doctrine of perfection is that of a wounded perfection, a scarred perfection, an imperfect perfection. This is why Paul, who understood broken bodies, was so conscious of weakness (*astheneia*: 1 Cor. 15.43; 2 Cor. 11.30; 12 5, 9ff.; 13.4; Gal. 4.13). Paul also said that God's weakness is stronger than human strength (1 Cor. 1.25), which could be translated, 'God's inability is stronger than human ability'; and he was comforted by God who did not reply to his prayer for strength, but told him that 'power is made perfect in weakness' (2 Cor. 12.9), or 'ability is made perfect in inability'.[24]

The Heavenly Session

The doctrine of the heavenly session refers to Christ seated in glory. It is based upon such passages as Mark 16.19, 'the Lord Jesus ... was taken up into heaven and sat down at the right hand of God', which is a late formulation, and upon several sayings of Jesus, such as, 'But from now on the Son of Man will be

---

24 I am grateful to Simon Hone, 'Those Who Are Blind: Some New Testament Uses of Impairment, Inability and Paradox', in Eiesland and Saliers (eds), *Human Disability*, Chapter 4, p. 88ff., for these insights.

seated at the right hand of the power of God' (Luke 22.69). The idea is prominent in the writings of Paul: 'he must reign until he has put all his enemies under his feet' (1 Cor. 15.25); and, 'it is Christ Jesus, who died, yes, who was raised, who is at the right hand of God, who indeed intercedes for us' (Rom. 8.34). From this last expression we learn that the idea is not only of Christ's sitting at the right hand of God as an exercise of authority and power, but is also a continuation of his mercy and grace on behalf of human beings. The heavenly session is also the heavenly intercession. This idea is a source of inspiration for Christian living: 'So if you have been raised with Christ, seek the things that are above, where Christ is, seated at the right hand of God' (Col. 3.1).[25]

The idea of the heavenly intercession leads naturally to the concept of Christ as High Priest. This is a central motif in the Letter to the Hebrews. As High Priest, the ascended and glorified Christ represents his earthly followers, and, just as a priest on earth offers sacrifices, so the great High Priest must have something to offer: 'he entered once for all into the Holy Place, not with the blood of goats and calves, but with his own blood' (Heb. 9.12). Thus, 'he entered into heaven itself, now to appear in the presence of God on our behalf' (Heb. 9.24).

Although the scars and wounds of the ascended Christ are not specifically mentioned in Hebrews, the idea of the High Priest presenting his blood and interceding does suggest the image. An important feature of the argument in Hebrews is that the High Priest was perfect (Heb. 7.26–28). This refers to the contrast between the repetition of the sacrifices offered by the earthly priests and the finality of the perfect sacrifice offered once for all (v. 28). Nevertheless, the High Priest remains a man who can 'sympathize with our weaknesses' and who 'in every respect has been tested as we are' (Heb. 4.15); 'he learned obedience through what he suffered' and, although he has been 'made perfect' and 'became the source of eternal salvation' (Heb. 5.8–9), he continues to present before God the evidence, so to speak, of his sufferings in the form of his blood.

---

25 Arthur J. Tait, *The Heavenly Session of Our Lord*, London: Robert Scott, 1912.

Adoration of the five wounds of Jesus became a feature of mystical contemplation in the Middle Ages, and the Cult of the Wound in the Side is to be found in the writings of Bonaventure (c. 1217–74) and others, although it was not theologically defined until the eighteenth century.[26] The stigmata, first received by Francis of Assisi (1181/2–1226) were always ambiguous in that it is unclear whether these replications of the five wounds were induced through meditation upon the crucifixion or upon the wounds of Christ the High Priest. This ambiguity became a matter of controversy with the Protestant Reformation in the sixteenth century.

The question was whether the Eucharist reproduced the actual body and blood of Christ. The reformers, in opposing transubstantiation, insisted that the real presence of the body of Christ could not be on earth, because it was already in heaven, at the right hand of God.[27] Moreover, it was argued that the sacrifice of Christ's death could not be repeated Sunday by Sunday since it had been offered by Christ once for all. This raised the question whether, when Christ showed himself to the Father, interceding for us, he was merely reminding the Father of the merits of his past sacrifice, or whether he was always engaged in a perpetual self-sacrifice.[28] One point of view, which is significant for a theology of disability, was that it was as a human being that Christ interceded before God. Theodore of Mopsuestia (c. 350–428) had taught that our human nature is already in heaven where Jesus Christ, in the body he received from the Virgin Mary, which was crucified, risen and ascended, represents us before God. Thus, the exultation of Christ is the exultation of the human.[29] Similarly, Jerome (c. 342–420) taught that 'Christ is said to intercede because He ever exhibits to the Father the manhood, which He took upon Him, as a pledge for

---

26 C. J. Walsh, 'Sacred Heart', in J. G. Davies (ed.), *A New Dictionary of Liturgy and Worship*, London: SCM Press, 1986, p. 473.

27 Christopher Elwood, *The Body Broken: The Calvinist Doctrine of the Eucharist, and the Symbolization of Power in Sixteenth Century France*, Oxford: Oxford University Press, 1999, pp. 36ff.

28 Tait, *Heavenly Session*, pp. 105–48.

29 Tait, *Heavenly Session*, p. 154.

us, and offers it, as the true and eternal High Priest.'[30] When the reformers of the sixteenth century sought to emphasize the transcendence of God by insisting that the body of Jesus Christ could not be on the altar because it was in heaven, it became natural to emphasize that the body of Christ still carried the marks of suffering. This emphasis entered into Protestant evangelical mysticism through Zinzendorf (1700–60) and his devotions to the wounds of Christ. From here it passed into the hymns of Charles Wesley as referred to above.

As far as we are concerned, these controversies are long since dead, but a significant point remains, and one that is hardly ever commented on in the interests of a theology of disability: the Man who sits at God's right hand is imperfect. The broken body on earth corresponds to the broken body in heaven. Moreover, the broken body on earth is to be found not only in the Eucharist, or the Lord's Supper, but also in the Church, which is the broken body of Christ, and in the broken body of suffering humanity. When people are hungry or thirsty, or naked, or sick, or in prison, it is Christ who suffers these things; and, because only a body can suffer thirst, hunger, nakedness, illness and imprisonment, it is not the Spirit but the body of Christ that suffers (Matt. 25.31–46).

We have found that, in addition to its mythological history of a perfection lost and to be regained, the Christian faith also expresses a profound and beautiful theology of brokenness.[31] Perhaps we could even say that a fundamental distinction can be made between churches and individual Christians: the theology of power, supremacy, uniqueness and prosperity is one form taken by the Christian faith today, and the theology of brokenness is its principal alternative. The theology of brokenness offers the Church a way of replacing the oppressive monolith of an unambiguous perfection with the rich and varied ambiguity of many forms of human brokenness.

---

30 Tait, *Heavenly Session*, p. 157.
31 This is developed by Jean Vanier in his theology undergirding the L'Arche communities of disabled people. Jean Vanier, *The Broken Body*, London: Darton, Longman and Todd, 1998.

Conclusions: Disability and the Mission of the Church

We have seen that when we start our thinking from the body of Christ, rather than from the image of God, we discover a theology of disability which is supported by various elements within the Christian faith. These include the implications of the fraction, that is, the breaking of the bread by the priest at the Eucharist, and the scarred and wounded body of Christ the King. The first of these symbols reminds us that brokenness lies at the heart of the paschal mystery and that the Church is united through brokenness. The second symbol reminds us that the Christian mythology, while it converges upon the perfection of a liberated cosmos, does not conform to the images of perfection found in our present culture, but witnesses to a range of patterns of perfection. At this point we encounter the Christian paradox of strength through weakness and life through death. The perfection of God is a perfection of vulnerability and of openness to pain. Part of the mission of the Church is to bear witness to the God of life by accepting many forms of human life and sharing in human vulnerability and pain. In this respect, part of the mission of disabled people is to become apostles of inclusion, witnesses of vulnerability and partners in pain.

9

'Sight to the Inly Blind'?

Attitudes to Blindness in the Hymnbooks

Part I: Evidence

John Merriott's (1780–1825) well-known missionary hymn 'Thou, whose almighty word' contains the following lines:

> Thou, who didst come to bring
> On thy redeeming wing
> Healing and sight,
> Health to the sick in mind,
> Sight to the inly blind,
> O now to all mankind
> Let there be light.[1]

But who are the inly blind? They are those who spiritually or psychologically possess the attributes of blindness. These are assumed to be insensitivity, ignorance and disbelief. The reference is not to those who are literally blind but to those who possess these characteristics inwardly. These negative implications could not be constructed unless blindness itself could really be described in this way, otherwise the analogy would lack credibility.

Such negative attitudes toward blindness are common in hymnbooks:

> Thy blessed unction from above
> Is comfort, life, and fire of love;

---

1 *Hymns Ancient & Modern Revised 1950*, no. 266.

Enable with perpetual light
The dullness of our blinded sight.[2]

It is the work of the Holy Spirit, to whom these lines are addressed, to restore human beings and to lift up our fallen, sinful nature, which is like blindness. Sometimes it is human mortality that is blind:

Awhile his mortal blindness
May miss God's loving kindness,
And grope in faithless strife:
But when life's day is over
Shall death's fair night discover
The fields of everlasting life.[3]

Charlotte Elliott's 1836 hymn 'Just as I am, without one plea' contains the verse:

Just as I am, poor, wretched, blind;
Sight, riches, healing of the mind,
Yea all I need, in thee to find,
O Lamb of God, I come.[4]

The thought is based upon Revelation 3.17: 'For you say, "I am rich, I have prospered, and I need nothing." You do not realize that you are wretched, pitiable, poor, blind, and naked.' The verse, like the hymn, attacks the complacency and self-deception of the Church or of those who have not responded to Christ, and blindness is associated with poverty, nakedness and wretchedness. The image of the blind beggar was as familiar to the early Victorians as it was to the early Christian communities.

---

2 Bishop John Cosin (1594–1672) adapted this hymn from the ninth or tenth-century Latin original for his *Collection of Private Devotions* (1627). *Hymns Ancient & Modern Revised 1950*, no. 157.

3 Translated by Robert Bridges (1844–1930) from the German of Paul Gerhardt (1607–76). *The New English Hymnal*, Norwich: Canterbury Press, 1986, no. 253.

4 Charlotte Elliott (1789–1871), *The New English Hymnal* revised 1996, no. 294.

A somewhat similar thought is expressed by the author of 'Father, hear Thy children's call':[5]

Blind, we pray that we may see,
Bound, we pray to be made free,
Stain'd, we pray for sanctity:
We beseech Thee, hear us.

Here, however, blindness is associated not so much with poverty and social exclusion as with inner bondage and moral impurity. Sometimes it is nature that is blind:

From the depths of nature's blindness,
From the hardening power of sin,
From all malice and unkindness,
From the pride that lurks within,
By Thy mercy,
O deliver us, good Lord.[6]

Sometimes it is the person belonging to another religious tradition. 'The heathen in his blindness/ Bows down to wood and stone.'[7] Sometimes it is the natural scientist:

Blind unbelief is sure to err,
And scan his work in vain;
God is his own interpreter,
And he will make it plain.[8]

Blindness is sometimes attributed to the nations in general, or perhaps to the nations that are the object of the Church's mission (Matt. 28.19).

---

5 *Hymns Ancient & Modern*, London, nd [1889], no. 465.
6 'Jesus, Lord of life and glory' by John Cummins (1795–1867), *The New English Hymnal* revised 1996, no. 68.
7 'From Greenland's icy mountains' by Bishop Reginald Heber (1783–1826), *Hymns Ancient & Modern Revised 1950*, no. 265.
8 'God moves in a mysterious way' by William Cowper (1731–1800), *Hymns Ancient & Modern Revised 1950*, no. 181.

> Sick, they ask for healing,
> Blind, they grope for day;
> Pour upon the nations
> Wisdom's loving ray.⁹

In the hymn 'Unchanging God, hear from eternal Heav'n' by the Reverend Samuel Stone (1839–1900),¹⁰ it is Judaism which is blind.

> These in soul-blindness now the far-away,
> These are not aliens, but Thy sons of yore,
> Oh, by Thy fatherhood, restore, restore!

Although people today are quick to deny that a connection can be assumed between sin and disability, the hymns sometimes suggest the contrary.

> Lord, remove our guilty blindness,
> Hallowed be Thy Name
> Show Thy Heart of loving kindness,
> Hallowed be Thy Name.
> By our heart's deep-felt contrition,
> By our mind's enlightened vision,
> By our will's complete submission,
> Hallowed be Thy Name.¹¹

Blindness is guilty but the enlightened mind has vision. The same point is made in another hymn by Timothy Rees, 'God is love: let heaven adore Him'.

> God is love: and though with blindness
> Sin afflicts the souls of men,

---

9 'Forward! Be our watchword' (1844) by Henry Alford (1810–71). Oremus hymnal, <http://www.oremus.org/hymnal>. The reference may be to the medical and educational aspects of the Church's foreign missions.

10 *Hymns Ancient & Modern* London nd [1889], no. 590, from the section 'Mission to the Jews'.

11 Timothy Rees (1874–1939) in *The Mirfield Mission Hymn Book*, Mirfield: The Community of the Resurrection [1916], no. 32.

God's eternal loving-kindness
Holds and guides them even then.[12]

Certainly, it is the soul not the body that is afflicted with blindness, but the singer is more likely to notice the connection between blindness and sin, while the allegory goes unremarked. In the hymn 'Spirit of God within me' by Timothy Dudley-Smith (1926–) the concept of blindness as an affliction is emphasized by attributing it to Satan.

> Spirit of truth within me,
>   Possess my thought and mind;
> Lighten anew the inward eye
>   By Satan rendered blind.[13]

Sometimes blindness is associated with a specific sin, such as pride; in the example that follows, the opposite of blindness is kindness.

> Drive out darkness from the heart,
>   Banish pride and blindness;
> Plant in every inward part
>   Truthfulness and kindness.[14]

The overwhelming influence in the hymns of blindness as in hymnody in general is, of course, the Bible. A famous example is the hymn 'I'll praise my Maker while I've breath', Isaac Watts' paraphrase of Psalm 146.

> The Lord gives eyesight to the blind;
>   The Lord supports the fainting mind;
> He sends the labouring conscience peace.[15]

---

12 *Mission Praise II*, London: Marshall Pickering, 1987, no. 368.
13 'Spirit of God within me' by Timothy Dudley-Smith (b. 1926) © Timothy Dudley-Smith in Europe and Africa. © Hope Publishing Company in USA. Extract reproduced by permission of Oxford University Press.
14 'Come, Lord, to our souls come down' by H. C. A. Gaunt (1902–83), Extract reproduced by permission of Oxford University Press.
15 Isaac Watts (1674–1748), *Mission Praise: combined words edition*, London: Marshall Pickering, 1990, no. 320.

The eschatological vision of the restoration of disabled people as found, for example, in Isaiah 35 is a popular subject. Charles Wesley writes:

> Hear him, ye deaf; his praise, ye dumb,
>   Your loosened tongues employ;
> Ye blind, behold your Saviour come;
>   And leap, ye lame, for joy![16]

The most important biblical references are to the healing ministry of Jesus Christ, and lame people are often linked with those with visual handicap.

> Thine arm, O Lord, in days of old,
> Was strong to heal and save;
> It triumph'd o'er disease and death,
> O'er darkness and the grave;
> To Thee they went, the blind, the dumb,
> The palsied and the lame,
> The leper with his tainted life,
> The sick with fever'd frame.[17]

> Why, what hath my Lord done?
> What makes this rage and spite?
> He made the lame to run,
> He gave the blind their sight.[18]

The theme is as popular today as ever, as in Geoffrey Marshall-Taylor's 'Go, tell it on the mountain':

> He reached out and touched them, the blind, the deaf, the lame;
> He spoke and listened gladly to anyone who came.[19]

---

16 'O for a thousand tongues to sing' by Charles Wesley (1707–88), *The New English Hymnal* revised 1996, no. 415. The verse is based upon Isa. 35.5.
17 E. H. Plumptre (1821–89), *Hymns Ancient & Modern*, no. 369.
18 Samuel Crossman (*c.* 1624–83), 'My song is love unknown', *Mission Praise*, London: Marshall Pickering, 1983, no. 160.
19 *Hymns & Psalms,* no. 135.

Sometimes the ministry of Christ is focused on his sermon in the synagogue in Nazareth. A well-known example is 'Hark the glad sound! The Saviour comes' by Philip Doddridge (1702–51).

> He comes to free the captive mind
> Where evil thoughts control;
> And for the darkness of the blind
> Gives light that makes them whole.[20]

In a more modern style, Alan Dale (1902–79) writes:

> He sent me to give the good news to the poor,
> Tell prisoners that they are prisoners no more,
> Tell blind people that they can see,
> And set the downtrodden free.[21]

Sometimes Jesus is described as continuing his healing ministry.

> Raise the fallen, cheer the faint,
>   Heal the sick, and lead the blind.[22]

The Church continues the ministry of Jesus.

> Jesus is the Name exalted
>   Over every other name;

---

[20] *Mission Praise: combined words edition*, no. 210. In a number of hymn-books including the 1889 and the 1950 editions of *Hymns Ancient & Modern* (no. 53) the hymn appears without the verse that refers to blindness. The original text, in *Hymns founded on Various Texts in the Holy Scriptures. By the late Reverend Philip Doddridge, D.D. Published from the Author's Manuscript*, 1755, reads:

He comes from thickest Films of Vice
To clear the mental Ray.
And on the Eye-Balls of the Blind
To pour celestial day.

Presumably the reference to balls struck a discordant note in the Victorian ear and was discarded. A number of modern versions re-introduce the thought of blindness but in a more refined way.

[21] 'God's spirit is in my heart', *Hymns & Psalms*, no. 315.

[22] 'Jesus lover of my Soul' by Charles Wesley, *Mission Praise*, 1983, no. 120.

In this Name, whene'er assaulted,
    We can put our foes to shame;
Strength to them who else had halted,
    Eyes to blind, and feet to lame.[23]

That we may care, as thou hast cared,
    For sick and lame, for deaf and blind,
And freely share, as thou hast shared,
    In all the sorrows of mankind.[24]

At first sight, the biblical references to blindness, including the very frequent allusions to the ministry of Jesus, do not seem to convey the same pejorative sense as the earlier cases we discussed. On closer examination, however, it is clear that the biblical attitude toward blindness is generally negative.[25] The healings of Jesus are not usually regarded today as mere miracles but are interpreted as symbolizing conversion from ignorance and unbelief to faith in Jesus.[26] 'I came into this world for judgement, so that those who do not see may see and those who do see may become blind' (John 9.39). Not to understand Jesus is to have poor sight. '[F]or those outside, everything comes in parables; in order that "they may indeed look, but not perceive"' (Mark 4.11–12). The unbelieving Pharisees are castigated by Jesus as being 'blind fools' (Matt. 23.17). When the Church continues the ministry of Jesus by offering medical and charitable services to blind people, it inherits not only his actions but also their meaning. Thus, the leper has not only a skin disease but a 'tainted life'; it is the captive mind that is set free by the gospel; and Christ 'for the darkness of the blind gives light that makes them whole'. When light is given to the inly blind they pass from ignorance into the

---

23 Tr. John Mason Neale (1818–66) from the fifteenth-century Latin original, *Hymns Ancient & Modern*, 1889, no. 179.
24 'Lord Christ, who on thy heart didst bear', Arnold Thomas (1848–1924), *Mission Praise II*, 394.
25 J. M. Hull, *In the Beginning There Was Darkness: A Blind Person's Conversations with the Bible*, London: SCM Press, 2001.
26 E. S. Johnson, 'Mark VIII: 22–26. The Blind Man from Bethsaida', *New Testament Studies* 25 (1979), pp. 370–83 and 'Mark X: 46–52: Blind Bartimaeus', *Catholic Biblical Quarterly* 40 (1978), pp. 191–204.

light of faith; what falls upon the eyes of blind people is not only light but 'celestial light'.

The metaphor of blindness touches nearly every Christian doctrine. In our created condition we are plunged in 'mortal blindness'; we confirm this through deliberate sin thus becoming wilfully blind; conversion restores our sight, and even eschatology is made more vivid through the metaphor of blindness.

> O quickly come, sure Light of all,
> For gloomy night broods o'er our way;
> And weakly souls begin to fall
> With weary watching for the day:
> O quickly come: for round Thy Throne
> No eye is blind, no night is known.[27]

In some hymns blindness becomes not so much a metaphor as an allegory of spiritual life.

> The very dimness of my sight
> Makes me secure;
> For, groping in my misty way,
> I feel His hand; I hear Him say,
> 'My help is sure.'
>
> I cannot read His future plans;
> But this I know:
> I have the smiling of His face,
> And all the refuge of His grace,
> While here below.
>
> Enough: this covers all my wants;
> And so I rest!
> For what I cannot, he can see,
> And in His care I saved shall be,
> For ever blest.[28]

---

[27] 'O quickly come, dread Judge of all', Lawrence Tuttiett (1825–97), *Hymns Ancient & Modern* [1889], no. 204.

[28] 'God holds the key of all unknown', Joseph Parker (1830–1902), *Mission Praise II*, no. 368.

The spiritual life is passive and dependent. Ignorance and illiteracy compel the believer to trust. This condition is described under the figure of blindness, or perhaps of visual impairment, although the inconsistency is seen in the fact that the believer, although groping in the darkness, can see the smiling face of God.[29] Writing like this reinforces the image of blind people as pathetically helpless while at the same time romanticizing the condition through suggesting that somehow the blind person displays desirable spiritual qualities.

Part II: Discussion

We have seen that reference to blindness in the hymns of the Church are frequent and always explicitly or implicitly negative. This feature is not unique to hymnody but is common in all forms of spoken and written English and in other languages. It would be interesting to know whether there is a language in which blindness is not used as a negative metaphor. Certainly in English it is so widespread and normal as to be almost invisible. As we saw in Chapter 4, in a recent collection of approximately 750 cases of the use of the word 'blind' in one of the quality daily newspapers,[30] literal and metaphorical use was evenly balanced. The striking fact is that almost all of the metaphorical examples were negative. 'He shows a blind disregard for the welfare of the country.' 'He struck out in blind fury.' 'She remains obstinately blind to the truth.' To be blind is to lack discrimination, to be ignorant, stubborn and insensitive. Our teachers speak of blind marking and our medical researchers of conducting a blind trial. In each case reference is made to the anonymity of the students or the unknown identity of the experimental group. Such expressions, however, reinforce the image of blindness as ignorance. It is not surprising that, when someone brought up in such a culture loses his or her sight, and all the unconscious negativity

---

29 I have discussed the way sighted theologians use the imagery of the divine face in Chapter 5 of this book.
30 Collated by me from the University of Birmingham COBUILD computerized word bank of English usage.

of blindness is turned in upon the self, there is a huge loss of self-esteem. Thus, the phenomenological loss of sight, serious enough in itself, is made worse by the oppressive language.

Within the Christian tradition we must face the fact that, far from liberating the language from such negative imaging, our Scriptures encourage it and our hymns reinforce it. The situation regarding people who are hard of hearing is pretty much the same.

Is this political correctness gone mad? There is no doubt that feminist and anti-racist critiques of language have brought about increased sensitivity to the way in which language is used to maintain the status of dominant groups, but the shadow of linguistic oppression is still cast upon disabled people. When 'political correctness' is used disparagingly by a dominant group, it becomes a defensive sneer. People in the marginalized group whose condition is stigmatized by the traditional language are justified in regarding the demand for political correctness as a call for emancipation.

The strange thing is that in most areas of disability the language has been more or less purged, at least in public. We no longer describe people with personality disorders as 'nut cases', and we rightly restrain our children if they call out 'spazzo' at a child who drops a ball. People suffering from impeded growth are no longer described as dwarves. We can best account for the survival of the negative metaphors of blindness and deafness on two grounds. First, these expressions are so deeply rooted in our language, and so widely used, that they have become inaudible. Even blind and deaf people seem often not to notice their implications. Second, the negative metaphors are supported by the Bible and are thus reinforced by piety. People whose reading of the Bible is respectful and devotional do not notice this aspect of the biblical language. If it is pointed out to them, they usually respond by saying that the language is metaphorical – which is just the problem.

When the attention of sighted church-goers is drawn to this issue, they tend to become apologetic about the use of candles, stained glass windows and metaphors of light. This, however, is quite unnecessary. As a blind person, I recognize that sighted people live in a world that is significantly different from my own. It is natural for them to rejoice in their world, and it is appropriate that religious truth should be conveyed to them in the language of their world. Nevertheless, they should not attack my world. They should not reinforce the significance of their own experience by denigrating mine. If sighted people wish to sing

> My eyes were closed; I could not see
> In Your marred visage any grace:
> But now the beauty of Your face
> In radiant vision dawns on me,

I have no objection, because they are using a metaphor that comes from within their own world – the closing of the eyes. However, this is not what W. T. Matson (1833–99) wrote, but: 'Lord I was blind: I could not see'. This becomes an attack on my world since blindness is now equated with unbelief.[31]

We must train ourselves to purify our language from unconscious traces of prejudice. The truth is that there is no such thing as spiritual blindness. There is spiritual insensitivity, stubbornness, ignorance and callousness, but when we refer to these qualities as being spiritual blindness we reinforce the prejudice, and collaborate in the continued marginalization of disabled people.

---

31 *Mission Praise: combined words edition*, no. 433. As a matter of fact, this hymn is a veritable litany of disablist metaphors, first criticizing blind people as unbelievers, deaf people as being unable to value the words of Jesus (v. 2), and people incapable of speech as being incapable of living for Jesus (v. 3). Perhaps a critic might point out that in verse 4 the memory of the dead is not held in reverence because they are regarded as unresponsive to the love of God, but, whatever we think about the dead, it is certain that the dead do not object and are not harmed by this negative stereotype as are the living communities of disabled people described in previous verses.

10

'Lord, I Was Deaf'

Images of Disability in the Hymnbooks

Introduction

In the previous chapter I studied some of the many references to blindness in hymns. I concluded that when the blind condition is treated as a symbol of sin and unbelief, a largely unconscious prejudice against blind people is reinforced. I suggested that the continued uncritical use of such hymns contributes to the marginalization and disempowerment of blind people in church and society. I remarked that 'the situation regarding people who are hard of hearing is pretty much the same', but I did not deal specifically with the imagery of deafness. In this chapter, I will present some examples of the metaphor of deafness in hymns, and I will add further examples of the use of blindness, leading to a discussion about the theological and ethical significance of this usage.

Deafness in the Hymnbooks

Let us start with the well-known hymn by William T. Matson (1833–99), the second and third verses of which go as follows

> Lord, I was deaf: I could not hear
> The thrilling music of Thy voice;
> But now I hear Thee and rejoice,
> And all Thine uttered words are dear.

> Lord, I was dumb: I could not speak
> The grace and glory of Thy name;
> But now, as touched with living flame,
> My lips Thine eager praises wake.[1]

It is estimated that there are about 50,000 people in the United Kingdom whose first, preferred language is British Sign Language (BSL).[2] This has been recognized by the UK government since 2003 as a language. While the UK does not have any official languages, in New Zealand sign language is the third official language of the country following English and Maori. It was once widely believed that signed languages, of which there are probably thousands in the world, were crude, concrete replications of spoken languages, but this view has long since been abandoned. It is now known that signed languages offer all the subtlety and variety of spoken language, both at the concrete, immediate level and at the most abstract and philosophical. In some respects, indeed, signed languages are superior to spoken ones. Speech is linear and mainly confined to sound, whereas signed language makes sophisticated use of space, movement and sequence; and the possibilities of simultaneity through the use of body and head movements as well as hands gives to signed language a remarkable richness which is indicated in the growing genre of signed poetry.[3] In addition to those whose preferred language is BSL, one must also recognize that about one person in seven in the UK has some degree of hardness of hearing, although retaining a preference for English as the medium of communication.

While Deaf[4] activists cooperate with other sections of the disabled community in campaigns for recognition and equality,

---

1 'Lord, I was blind: I could not see', *Mission Praise: combined words edition*, London: Marshall Pickering, 1990, no. 433.

2 The Royal Association for Deaf People, <http://www.royaldeaf.org.uk/page.php?id=100177>.

3 R. Sutton-Spence, 'Aspects of BSL Poetry: A Social and Linguistic Analysis of the Poetry of Dorothy Miles', *Sign Language and Linguistics* 3:1 (2000), pp. 79–100, <http://www.ingentaconnect.com/content/jbp/sll/2000/00000003/00000001/art00004>.

4 In the disability literature, Deaf with a capital often refers to people whose preferred communication is sign language, while deaf with a lower case refers to hearing loss in general.

many do not regard deafness as a disability but as a feature of a persecuted linguistic minority. There are cases, mostly in small or isolated communities with a large number of Deaf people, where some form of signing has become general throughout the community. In such situations attention is seldom drawn to the inability to hear or speak as a significant characteristic of someone.[5] Moreover, study of the spirituality, religious life and theology of Deaf communities has revealed distinct characteristics, often involving sophisticated perceptions and sensitivities that may not be present in speaking and hearing communities.[6]

However, there is little trace of this respect for deaf culture in the hymnbooks. For example, no. 85 in *Hymns Ancient & Modern* is a seventeenth-century hymn first published in English in 1839 and intended for use during evensong. It is a meditation on John 1.5, 'The light shineth in the darkness and the darkness comprehended it not'. Sensory deprivation is used to illustrate a negative attitude towards Judaism.

> Now heaven's growing light is manifest
> Through Judah's land which in the darkness lies;
> But they have steel'd their breast,
> And closed their earth bound eyes.
>
> Now signs of present Godhead teem around,
> The dead are raised, feet to the lame are given,
> The dumb a tongue hath found,
> The blind man sees the heaven.
>
> But Israel hath become blind, deaf and dead ...[7]

Most of the references to deafness in hymns can be traced back to the influence of the Bible. This appears in three ways, the most important of which is the healing miracles of Jesus.

---

5 Nora Ellen Groce, *Everyone Here Spoke Sign Language: Hereditary Deafness on Martha's Vineyard*, London: Harvard University Press, 1985.

6 Wayne Morris, *Theology without Words: Theology in the Deaf Community*, Aldershot: Ashgate, 2008.

7 *Hymns Ancient & Modern: Historical Edition*, London: William Clowes, 1909, p. 115.

> To Thee they went, the deaf, the dumb,
> The palsied and the lame.
> The beggar with his sightless eyes,
> The sick with fevered frame.[8]

The second biblical influence is eschatological hope. When the Kingdom of God comes in its fullness, there will be no more sicknesses and impairments, as is foretold in Isaiah 35.5, 6: 'Then the eyes of the blind shall be opened, and the ears of the deaf unstopped; then the lame shall leap like a deer, and the tongue of the speechless sing for joy.'

> Surely he cometh and a thousand voices
> Shout to the saints, and to the deaf are dumb;
> Surely he cometh and the earth rejoices,
> Glad in his coming who hath sworn: I come![9]

This presumably means that unbelievers, who are described as being deaf and dumb, will not be aware of the triumphant voices announcing the second coming of Christ. The well-known hymn by Graham Kendrick takes up a similar eschatological theme but more positively.

> He comes the broken hearts to heal
> The prisoners to free.
> The deaf shall hear, the lame shall dance,
> The blind shall see.
> ...
> Make way! (Make way!)
> And let his kingdom in.[10]

Whenever Jesus Christ is preached his earthly miracles are symbolically repeated, and at the announcement of the gospel disabilities flee away.

---

8 E. H. Plumptre (1821–91), 'Thine arm, O Lord, in days of old', *Common Praise*, Norwich: Canterbury Press, 2000, no. 347.

9 F. W. H. Myers (1343–1901), 'Hark what a sound and too divine for hearing', *Common Praise*, no 28, v. 2.

10 Graham Kendrick (1950–), 'Make way! Make way!', *Songs of Fellowship*, Eastbourne: Kingsway Music, 1998, no. 384.

> Hear Him, ye deaf; His praise, ye dumb,
> Your loosen'd tongues employ,
> Ye blind, behold your saviour come
> And leap, ye lame, for joy![11]

The third biblical influence that can sometimes be detected is the God of the Bible depicted as a perfect human being with no trace of impairment.

> Lord, we are few, but Thou art near,
> Nor short Thine arm, nor deaf Thine ear;
> O rend the heav'ns, come quickly down,
> And make a thousand hearts Thine own.[12]

In many hymns the reference is not so much to hearing impairment as to the refusal to listen on the part of people with hearing, a refusal for which they may be regarded as morally culpable. Many hymns also refer to hearing people as being unable to hear, or unable to hear clearly because of a spiritual incapacity for which they may or may not be responsible.

> May Thy dread voice around,
> Thou harbinger of light,
> On our dull ears still sound,
> Lest here we sleep in night.[13]

> Give us the tongues to speak,
> In every time and place,
> To rich and poor, to strong and weak,
> The word of love and grace.
> Enable us to hear
> The words that others bring,

---

[11] Charles Wesley (1707–88), 'O for a thousand tongues to sing', *The New English Hymnal* revised 1996, no. 415, v. 5.

[12] William Cowper (1731–1800), 'Jesus, where'er thy people meet', *Common Praise*, no. 492, v. 5. The reference is to Isaiah 59.1. On the question of God as a normal or supernormal human being see Chapter 5 of the present volume.

[13] C. Coffin (1676-1749), tr. I. Williams in 1839, 'Lo! from the desert homes', *Hymns Ancient & Modern Revised 1950*, no. 552.

Interpreting with open ear
The special song they sing.[14]

The contrast between the literally Deaf who are nevertheless open to religious experience and the literally hearing who nevertheless refuse to respond to faith is made specific in John Keble's poem or hymn for the 12th Sunday after Trinity:

The deaf may hear the saviour's voice
The fettered tongue its chain may break
But the deaf heart, the dumb by choice,
The laggard soul that waits
The guilt that scorns to be forgiven,
These baffle e'en the bells of heaven.[15]

In English as in most languages to hear is to pay attention, to listen with understanding and receptivity. A parent might say to a disobedient child, 'You are not to do that! Do you hear me?' and when a congregation prays, 'O Lord hear our prayer and let our cry come unto Thee,' it is a plea for the divine response. There is a sliding scale, from explicit references to members of the Deaf community – although these are also intended in a metaphorical sense – to such expressions as 'She was deaf to my entreaty', where the reference is to a refusal to respond, and to such expressions as Antony's asking the Romans to lend him their ears, and the prayer 'O give me Samuel's ear'.[16] When Jesus said 'If you have ears to hear, then hear' there was no negative reference to Deaf people. But surely, in that case, we might reflect, no negative reference to the literally deaf is intended in any of these hymns?

There may be unintended consequences of both speech and action, and when these are realized by the speaker or the actor, the nature of the consequences comes to the foreground of intention and demands choice. That deaf people have been marginalized,

---

14 Michael Forster (1946–), 'Come, Holy Spirit, come!', *Common Praise*, no. 179, v. 4.
15 John Keble, *The Christian Year*, London, 1827.
16 James Drummond Burns (1823–64), 'Hush'd was the evening hymn', *Mission Praise: combined words edition*, no. 253.

patronized, excluded and persecuted is a matter of history, and that history is not over yet. Therefore we have to look for the causes or contributory factors that have built up or sustained those attitudes. There can be no doubt that the use of deafness as a metaphor for incomprehension and disobedience at least suggests a negative attitude on the part of society and to some extent sustains it, whether consciously or not. After all, you might as well say that those who speak and understand only French are inattentive, stubborn and disobedient when given orders in English! It is simply that they don't speak English, and neither do many of those whose preferred life-long language is BSL. This says nothing about their intelligence, their inter-personal skills or their religious sensitivity, and the same is true, of course, of people who have lost part or most of their hearing later in life, whether or not they use BSL. So when church tradition whether in Scripture or in hymns speaks of those who refuse to pay attention to the Christian message or to respond to the appeal of Christ as being hard of hearing or deaf, a link is set up, whether asserted or merely taken for granted, between those attributes and people in the deaf community.

The problem is complicated by the fact that one cannot voluntarily close one's ears. We have eyelids but not earflaps. We can close our eyes to a situation, meaning that we refuse to take note of it, but such a figure of speech would be inappropriate for the sense of hearing. We would not normally or naturally say that someone closed their ears to an appeal for help; we would say that the person had refused to listen or, to put it more poetically, was 'dull of hearing'. When we say 'he was deaf to their entreaties' we mean no more than that he failed to hear or respond to certain sounds just as a deaf person might have done. To say that Deaf people do not respond to spoken language is, at one level, merely to remark that Deaf people have their own form of communication; but, on the other hand, these expressions almost always carry with them a critical or negative meaning. We criticize someone for being deaf to an appeal because we believe that there should have been a response and that the person was responsible for not responding, but Deaf people are not responsible for not responding to spoken appeals.

We have now reached a position where we can establish a criterion for the unacceptable use of the metaphors taken from the sense of hearing. The question we must ask is whether the expression, intentionally or not, is pejorative. Are deaf people, whether literally or metaphorically, being blamed or having moral, spiritual or character defects attributed to them, directly or by inference? In short, when John Keble writes,

> Come, Lord, come wisdom, love and power,
> Open our ears to hear.
> Let us not miss the accepted hour:
> Save, Lord, by love or fear,[17]

there is no disparaging reference to members of the deaf community. When Charles Wesley, on the other hand, writes,

> Hear Him, ye deaf, His praise, ye dumb,
> Your loosen'd tongues employ,[18]

there is clearly an implication that those who do not respond to the Christian message because of insensitivity or disobedience are like members of the Deaf community. To say this is not to criticize Charles Wesley. He had no way of knowing about the sophistication of British Sign Language, and he probably had no idea that there is a spirituality and theology of Deaf people which might be as profound as that found in the speaking community. We today, however, do know or should know these things and should be able to remove those elements in our tradition that continue to collaborate with this ancient, ignorant prejudice.

Blindness in the Hymnbooks

Let us now return to the more frequent occurrence of visual metaphorical language. When J. M. Neale translates a hymn from the

---

17 John Keble (1792–1866), 'When God of old came down from heaven', *Common Praise*, no. 199, v. 7.
18 From the hymn 'O for a thousand tongues to sing', *The New English Hymnal* revised 1996, no. 415. The verse is based upon Isa. 35.5.

late evening service of the Orthodox Church, there is no hint of a disparaging attitude towards blind people.

> Lord, that in death I sleep not
> And lest my foe should say
> 'I have prevailed against him,'
> Lighten mine eyes I pray:
> O, Jesu, keep me in Thy sight
> And guard me through the coming night.[19]

Similarly, when Bishop James Russel Woodford (1820–85) speaks of 'our darkened sight' the context shows that he is thinking of the contrast between day and night, or perhaps a sky overcast with heavy clouds and a clear sky: there is no hint of a negative allusion to blind people.

> 'Til from our darkened sight
>   The cloud shall pass away.
> And on the cleansed soul shall burst
>   The everlasting day.[20]

References to 'dim eyes' are more ambiguous. Here the reference is not to the weather, or to the rotation of the earth, but to people with poor sight.

> Yet when Thine Easter-news was spread,
> 'Mid all its light, his eyes were dim.[21]

The reference is to St Thomas, and although the Gospel of John describes him as a stout unbeliever who demands visual and tactile proof of the resurrection, there is nothing in the story to suggest that he had any problems with his eyesight. 'Dim eyes' has become a metaphor for his lack of faith.

---

19 Tr. Dr J. M. Neale, 'The day is past and over', *Hymns Ancient & Modern: Historical Edition*, no. 19.
20 James Russel Woodford (1820–85), 'Within the Father's house', *Hymns Ancient & Modern: Historical Edition*, no. 87, v. 6.
21 William Bright (1824–1901), 'How oft O Lord, Thy face hath shone', *Hymns Ancient & Modern: Historical Edition*, no. 226.

IMAGES OF DISABILITY IN THE HYMNBOOKS

Another ambiguous example comes from the well-known hymn 'Holy, holy, holy'. Verse 3 reads:

Holy! Holy! Holy! Though the darkness hide thee,
Though the eye of sinful man Thy glory may not see ...[22]

It is one thing to say that God dwells in darkness but it is another thing to claim that it is because of sin one cannot see. No doubt it is sin that prevents human beings from becoming aware of the divine glory, but, as one who on many occasions has been asked about the alleged sin that brought about my blindness, I cannot be comfortable with this line.[23]

I have a similar sense of slight discomfort with the words in the well-known hymn 'Break Thou the bread of life'. The third verse goes:

O send Thy spirit, Lord, now unto me,
That he may touch my eyes, and make me see:
Show me the truth concealed within Thy word,
And in Thy book revealed I see Thee, Lord.[24]

This is a prayer for understanding based upon the sense of sight. The reference to being made to see by the touching of the eyes brings the metaphor close to the idea of blindness, reminiscent as it is of the miracle of the man born blind in John 9.

There are many cases, however, where the metaphor of blindness is used less ambiguously to describe sinful, unbelieving or unresponsive people.

Thou knowest what we are, how frail and blind,
Thou still rememb'rest that we are but dust:
Like as a Father pitieth, Thou art kind ...[25]

---

22 Reginald Heber (1783–1826), 'Holy, holy, holy! Lord God Almighty!', *Common Praise*, no. 202, v. 3.
23 For examples see my *In the Beginning There Was Darkness: A Blind Person's Conversations with the Bible*, London: SCM Press, 2001, pp. 49–52.
24 Mary Lathbury (1841–1913) and Alexander Groves (1842–1909), 'Break Thou the bread of Life', *Common Praise*, no. 286, v. 3.
25 Ernest Edward Dugmore (1843–1925), 'Almighty Father, Unoriginate', *Hymns Ancient & Modern: Historical Edition*, no. 34, v. 5.

In a hymn written in 1899 for the war in South Africa blindness is identified with careless living. This is odd, since one of the most obvious features of living as a blind person is that one has to be so careful about everything.

> Spare us, good Lord! If just the strife
> Yet still from guilt we are not free;
> Forgive our blind and careless life,
> Our oft forgetfulness of Thee.[26]

As with deafness, many references to blindness in the hymn-books are influenced by the miracles of Jesus.

> Pass me not, O mighty Spirit!
> Thou canst make the blind to see;
> Witnesser of Jesu's merit
> Speak the word of power to me –
> Even me.[27]

Another example is the hymn by Tommy Walker from 1995:

> Only you are the Author of life
> Only you can bring the blind their sight
> Only you are called Prince of Peace.[28]

Other hymns are influenced by the sermon preached by Jesus at Nazareth. An example is the popular and beautiful hymn from the Iona community.

> Will you let the blinded see
> If I but call your name?
> Will you set the prisoners free
> And never be the same?[29]

---

26 Somerset Corry Lowry (1855–1932), 'Lord, while afar our brothers fight', *Hymns Ancient & Modern: Historical Edition*, no. 519.

27 Elizabeth Codner (1824–1919), 'Lord, I hear of showers of blessing', *Hymns Ancient & Modern: Historical Edition*, no. 593.

28 Tommy Walker, 'I will give you praise', *Songs of Fellowship*, no. 270.

29 John Bell (1949–) and Graham Maule (1958–), 'Will you come and follow me if I but call your name?', *Common Praise*, no. 622, v. 3.

The same influence is probably to be seen in the hymn by C. A. Callington (1872–1955), although there are also traces of the commission given to Paul following his brief loss of sight.

> Tell the praise of him who called you
> Out of darkness into light,
> Broke the fetters that enthralled you,
> Gave you freedom, peace and sight.[30]

Another influence is Revelation 3.17:

> We are wretched, cold and naked,
> Needing all things, poor and blind;
> Thou hast raiment, riches, healing,
> Meet for body, soul, and mind.[31]

Most descriptions of blindness in the hymns refer to personal conversion or to the transforming power of Christian faith.

> I was once in darkness, now my eyes can see,
> I was lost but Jesus sought and found me.[32]

> Once I was blind,
> Yet believed I saw everything
> Proud in my ways
> Yet a fool in my heart.[33]

In the light of Matthew 23.17, where Jesus is described as having spoken of blind fools, the connection in this hymn between blindness and foolishness is regrettable.

Perhaps the most striking cases are those where the metaphor of blindness is used to describe not one's own shortcomings but those of others. So, in 1936, Percy Dearmer wrote:

---

30 C. A. Callington (1872–1955), 'Ye that know the Lord is gracious', *Common Praise*, no. 628, v. 3.
31 August Blair Donaldson (1841–1903), 'Glory to the first-begotten', *Hymns Ancient & Modern: Historical Edition*, no. 629.
32 Joan Parsons, 'I once was in darkness', *Songs of Fellowship*, no. 263.
33 Stuart Townend, 'I will sing of the lamb', *Songs of Fellowship*, no. 856, v. 3.

O, free the world from blindness,
and fill the world with kindness,
Give sinners resurrection,
bring striving to perfection.[34]

In a similar vein, Chris Cartwright in 1991 writes:

Interceding for a nation
That is dying, lost and blind,
Let us see them with the eyes of Christ.[35]

In 1996, Lex Loizides sings:

Our hearts were turned away,
But then the light of Christ broke in
And made us live again.
And if you can heal our blindness,
You can save our nation too.[36]

Occasionally, the hymn writers show an awareness that it may be religion itself that will be the problem: 'Let not our worship blind us to the claims of love.'[37]

Further Thoughts about the Criterion

Before we began to refer to the metaphor of sight and blindness we had arrived at a discriminating criterion. This was to ask ourselves if the metaphor suggested a disparaging comparison with groups of disabled people. I would now like to suggest a more searching rationale for this. If sighted and hearing people

---

34 Percy Dearmer (1867–1936), 'A brighter dawn is breaking', *Common Praise*, no. 135, v. 3.
35 Chris Cartwright, 'From your throne, O Lord', *Songs of Fellowship*, no. 725.
36 Lex Loizides, 'We stand together before our saviour', *Songs of Fellowship*, no. 1103.
37 George B. Caird, 'Almighty Father, who for us thy Son didst give', *Common Praise*, no. 374, v. 4.

use the imagery of light and sound to express their experiences in the world they inhabit, that is natural and inevitable. However, if able-bodied people make disparaging allusions to people who have very different experiences this may not only betray ignorance of those ways of life and is discourteous, but may reinforce a prejudice against disabled people that will in turn give credibility to the view that the Christian faith does not offer answers to the search for equal opportunities: it may actually be part of the problem. In other words, when we consider the sliding scale of metaphors, from those that refer explicitly to various impaired states through to those that merely use the various ideas of light and sound, sight and speech, we should distinguish between those that speak to our own world, the one we know and experience, and those that refer negatively to other people's worlds of which we have no first-hand experience.

In saying this, I do not overlook the fact that there may be hymn writers who are themselves blind yet continue to use disparaging metaphors of their own condition. This is to be explained by the combination of a piety that does not adopt a critical stance towards the tradition, and immersion in the assumptions of a society in which the inferiority and the marginalization of disabled people were simply taken for granted.

In the light of our new principle it is possible to comment on the situation of people with other impairments such as those who use wheelchairs for mobility. Biblical precedent such as the eschatological hope expressed in Isaiah 35.5 and some of the miracles in the Gospels do encourage the hymn writers to refer to lame people. Lameness can be used as a disparaging metaphor for sin. Such expressions are as unacceptable as the explicitly pejorative references to blind and deaf people. Merely referring to standing up, however, comes into the category of speaking of the body's symbolism which is natural to those who have legs and can use them. A wheelchair user should no more object to 'Stand up and bless the Lord, ye people of His choice'[38] than I as a blind person have any right to object to 'The Lord is my

---

38 James Montgomery (1771–1854), 'Stand up and bless the Lord', *Mission Praise: combined words edition*, no. 615.

light, my strength and my salvation'. True, the Lord is not my light, because I have no light sensation, and wheelchair users cannot respond to the invitation to stand up in the presence of the Lord.[39] However, just as able-bodied people should not thrust the demands of their experience upon others, so people with impairments should not demand that able-bodied worlds should conform to theirs. The principle is to rejoice in your own world without making disparaging remarks or setting unreasonable limits upon the natural life-worlds of others.

A limited range of disabilities are referred to in the hymn-books. These are usually those that find a symbolic place within the vocabulary of the Bible: blindness, deafness, being lame or having leprosy. We referred earlier to the hymn 'Thine arm O Lord, in days of old', quoting the line 'the beggar with his sightless eyes'. This replaced the line, found in the older version, 'the leper with his tainted life', which has not reappeared in that particular hymn since about 1950.[40] References to diseases such as AIDS and cancer are rarely if ever found in hymns, partly because they are contemporary conditions, and partly because they are not referred to in the Bible.

Bodily Metaphors

This discussion raises questions about the whole use of metaphors based upon the human body. Such language is inevitable, depending upon the kind of body you are born with, and without it language would become very colourless. We could not speak at all without metaphor and most of our metaphors are based upon very early body experience.[41] When we say such

---

39 I am referring to the words of hymns not to the conduct of public worship. There is a growing awareness of diversity in congregations, and increasingly leaders of worship are using such expressions as 'If you normally stand then please stand now' or 'If you would like to stand please do so', which respect the varieties of physical posture that may be convenient for the worshippers.

40 Edward Hayes Plumptre (1821–91), 'Thine arm, O Lord, in days of old', *Hymns Ancient & Modern: Historical Edition*, no. 552.

41 Mark Johnson, *The Body in the Mind: The Bodily Basis of Meaning, Imagination and Reason*, Chicago: University of Chicago Press, 1990.

things as 'I can't quite follow you', 'We seem to have gone about as far as we can with this discussion', 'At this point our thought encounters an obstacle', and so on, we are using language that originates in bodily life in the world. Rooted in our earliest infancy, such expressions not only make language more meaningful but become more or less invisible as metaphors. If we were spirits, unconscious of pain, obstacles, hunger or death, and if we communicated by spiritual intuition without the use of hands, lips and tongues, we might be able to manage without such metaphors, but then we would no longer be human. The bodily experience of most human beings takes place in a world in which there is light and darkness, sound and silence, arms and legs, mobility and music, but modern understandings of human rights demand that the plurality of human worlds should be recognized. This demand bites deeply (another body metaphor) into a tradition that has not found it easy to recognize plurality. The very idea that some day in the future the diversity of human persons will converge upon the experience of the majority illustrates this difficulty. The concept of a homogeneous perfection against which diversity is considered to be imperfect encourages the marginalization of minority groups. Perhaps it will be said that able-bodied people, who are in the majority, are fully justified in speaking negatively of blindness and deafness. After all, it might be said, would not the deaf prefer to hear and the blind to see?

In the first place, Deaf culture is becoming increasingly autonomous. It cannot be assumed that deaf people would prefer to hear; the assumption would be considered by many in the Deaf world as part of the arrogance typical of a powerful majority. In the case of blind people, with their greater loss of independent movement, and the loss of so much visual beauty, it might be more unusual to find blind people who would not prefer to see.[42] Be this as it may, it does not justify the assumption or the claim being made by sighted people. The situation is rather

---

[42] Unusual, but not unknown: Oliver Sacks describes the case of Virgil, a blind man from Kentucky who was deeply disorientated and depressed when sight was restored to him. There are other reports of such cases. Oliver Sacks, *An Anthropologist on Mars*, London: Picador, 1995, pp. 102-44.

similar to the relationship between the rich and the poor. It may be that the poor are blessed, but it is not the place of the rich to say so. Moreover, sometimes the disparagement of presumably less desirable states leaves an uneasy feeling (another body metaphor) that it springs from a nervousness about the loss of a normality. Anyone can lose sight or hearing at almost any time. Normality is as temporary and as fragile as blindness and deafness appear to be undesirable. So let not the strong people glory in their strength, nor the normal in their normality, nor the wise in their wisdom, but let the one who glories, glory in the Lord. Certainly, there are many Christian disabled people whose experience testifies that whether they live or die, whether they see or not, whether in wheelchairs or not, they live in the hands of God – and that is another bodily metaphor.

Conclusions

Negative metaphors of various disabilities are not only found in the hymnbooks and the Bible, but are common in the media and in everyday speech. Perhaps they will become less common in a more enlightened community. We will always have to face the fact that much of the classical literature of the world embodies such negativity. What are we to say, for example, of the use of literal blindness as a metaphor in Shakespeare's *King Lear*? It seems reasonable to hope that, just as the presence of anti-Semitism in *The Merchant of Venice* and misogynist views in *The Taming of the Shrew* present problems for contemporary producers, so references to *The Hunchback of Notre Dame* and the blindness of Gloucester will increasingly be regarded as traces of archaic prejudice. Will the same thing happen to the Bible or will enough Christians be inspired by its generally redemptive message to distance themselves and others from its lesser negative motifs? The greatness of Shakespeare will survive the realization of the presence of some less acceptable attitudes, and the same is true of the spiritual majesty of the Bible.

In view of the fact that the Christian faith has so much potential for human liberation it is sad and puzzling to see that the realization and implementation of this has taken many centuries. Although the biblical doctrines of creation and redemption surely imply that no human being should own another one as his or her property, parts of the Bible are fairly complacent towards the institution of slavery. For centuries it was in the interest of the wealthy and powerful to collaborate with the convenience of slavery, and this is still the case in some respects today. Similarly, the equal creation of men and women and the equality of their calling in the Christian community should have enabled those who were newly created in the image of Christ to overcome the patriarchal prejudice that is found in so much of the Bible, but it did not always do so. The recognition that disabled people are not subhuman, and that much of what we call disability is caused not by their impairment as such but by the attitudes and environment of the surrounding society, has also been very slow to mature. The miracles of Jesus, which might perhaps have encouraged the inclusion of disabled people in the community have seldom been interpreted in this way.[43] The miracles certainly encouraged a mission of healing but this often took the form of isolation and exclusion. Taken literally, the miracles have encouraged the view that there is no real place for disabled people among the disciples of Jesus;[44] taken symbolically they have led to the negativity that we have been discussing. The liberation offered by Jesus in his death and resurrection was not enough to overcome the negative imagery of the Bible.

These are sad reflections, but not hopeless ones. To use two more bodily metaphors, the night is far spent but the morning is at hand. Many contemporary hymnbooks have been careful to remove traces of imperialism and patriarchy. Sensitivity towards the negative images of disabled people has hardly begun, but it is not impossible that this will be the next wave of reform.

---

43 Graham W. Monteith, *Deconstructing Miracles: From Thoughtless Indifference to Honouring Disabled People*, Glasgow: Covenanters Press, 2005.

44 John M. Hull, 'Could a Blind Person Have Been a Disciple of Jesus?', *Ministerial Formation* [World Council of Churches Education and Ecumenical Formation] 92 (2001), pp. 20–1, <http://www.johnmhull.biz/Could%20a%20blind%20person.html>.

Let us conclude with one final example, perhaps the best-known and best-loved hymn in which a negative image of blindness is conveyed.

> Amazing grace –
> how sweet the sound –
> That saved a wretch like me!
> I once was lost, but now am found,
> Was blind, but now I see.[45]

I would like to suggest a slightly altered version.

> Amazing grace that set me free
> And brought me to the light.
> I once was blind but now I see,
> Was black but now I'm white.

Most people today would, I imagine, find the last line objectionable. So why not the second last line? A reformed version followed:

> Amazing grace, how sweet the sound
> That saved a wretch like me!
> I once was lost, but now am found,
> Was bound, but now I'm free.

---

45 John Newton (1725–1807), 'Amazing Grace', *Mission Praise: combined words edition*, no. 31.

11

Teaching as a Trans-world Activity

We normally assume that we are conscious of our passions. We speak of being swept away by passion, of being overwhelmed, of someone who has a passion for art, or who breaks out into a passionate defence of someone. Moments of passion are moments of intense emotional absorption, when we are aware of little else but the passion itself. Indeed, in many such moments we forget ourselves. We even explain our behaviour by saying 'I quite forgot myself'. In a strange way, passion tends towards self-forgetfulness.

Passion is the emotional realization of intense desire, but we are aware of that which excites our passion, not of ourselves. Desire is not always conscious of desiring, but only of that which is desired.

Are there then desires so deep, so all-pervading that we are unaware of them? Attention is focused by contrast – the distinction between what is and is not relevant, between information and background noise, between presence and absence. But if there were a desire so perennial, so unwavering in its persistence, would we be unaware of it? Would it so completely fill the horizon of consciousness that no contrast would draw it to our attention?

The Desire to See

The Oxford philosopher Brian Magee has suggested that sight has this characteristic. He speaks of 'this almost ungovernable lust' to see, such a powerful desire that it can only be satisfied by continual seeing.[1] Magee suggests that 'it is the feeding of this almost ungovernable craving that constitutes the ongoing pleasure of sight'. He remarks that this is something of which most people are quite unaware, although they live continually in it. We can, he suggests, live in an all-encompassing desire so natural to us that we become unaware of it. Magee contrasts the avidity to see with the character of our desire to hear. 'This has no parallel with the senses of hearing, taste or smell: we are under no slavish compulsion to be hearing sounds all the time, or tasting tastes, or smelling smells.'[2] Magee suggests that the desire to hear is perhaps not comparable with the desire to see, although the need to touch and feel may be somewhat similar. There is the pleasure of near sensation, the delight of being in a sensuate body, the difficulty most people have in imagining what it would be like to be without bodily sensation, to be paralysed from the neck down, to become entirely numb. The world of feeling is, perhaps, so basic that it is tantamount to the desire for life itself – the fundamental pleasures of breathing, of the heart-throb.

The pleasure of seeing is highlighted by the fact that for sighted people seeing is virtually the same as consciousness. For most of the time, to be conscious is to have one's eyes open, and thus to see. There are exceptions: sighted people tend to close their eyes for a moment when they are deep in thought, or in order to concentrate on music, or when kissing. Usually, however, we return to consciousness from sleep with the opening of our eyes, and we prepare for sleep as our eyelids become heavy.

If it is true that for sighted people seeing is such a basic part of the mainly unconscious pleasures of life, if it is really coextensive with existence as such, it would be difficult to imagine another form of life. This is why McGee concludes his discussion by saying:

> [I]t seems to me that most people's perception of the world, of things, of reality including other people is so heavily weighted

---

[1] B. Magee and M. Milligan, *On Blindness: Letters Between Bryan Magee and Martin Milligan*, Oxford: Oxford University Press, 1995, p. 104.

[2] Magee and Milligan, *On Blindness*, p. 105.

with vision-derived content, that if that were removed, what was left would seem to them to be so drastically impoverished as to be scarcely any longer a world.³

From Normality to Totality

In the light of the fundamental character of the sighted person's existence in the world, it is inevitable that there is a tendency to believe that our experience of the world is equivalent to the world. We tend to mistake our experience of reality for reality itself.⁴ Since our experience is of a totality,

> we proceed as if what this leaves out cannot really make all that much difference, as if total reality cannot but correspond pretty well to the experience we have of it, and therefore anything we lack must be something we can compensate for fully or almost fully. Most people cannot help believing in their experience, 'and that outside of this there is nothing and cannot be anything'.⁵

Sight is the basis of a whole world and, by a natural cognitive inference, the wholeness turns into a totality. The wholeness of the sighted world becomes unconscious because there is no contrast, and it becomes total because the mere possibility of contrast is difficult to contemplate. The fundamental character of sight establishes itself as a fundamentalism, which reigns all the more powerfully because those who live in it are unaware of it. I do not, of course, mean that sighted people do not know they are sighted. I am suggesting that very few sighted people realize the degree to which the world in which they live is the projection of their sighted bodies. The sighted world becomes absolute because there is nothing else alongside it which can relativize it. It is thus highly likely, perhaps inevitable, that the sighted world will not comprehend sightlessness. To comprehend it would be

---

3 Magee and Milligan, *On Blindness*, p. 106.
4 Magee and Milligan, *On Blindness*, p. 19.
5 Magee and Milligan, *On Blindness*, pp. 99–100.

to relativize one's own sighted experience, to abandon the confident and unselfconscious sense of absolute normality which brings the assurance and power of living.

How then do sighted people regard sightless people? Those without sight are usually thought of as being excluded not merely from *a* world but from *the* world. A deficiency model of blindness is the tribute sighted people pay to their own normality. But a deficiency model is based upon exclusion, and exclusion if it is charitably inclined must seek for a benevolent inclusion, and must approach the other with a surplus of compassion, in view of the fact that the blind person, being excluded from the world, has no world.

The sighted world thus approaches its own limits with a compassion that borders upon horror. The fear is the fear of being without the basis of life. The natural desire of the healthily normal to reinstate its possession of normality is challenged by horror when its limit is perceived. There is a horror of deep darkness from which the light instinctively recoils. One of the ways we handle horror is by turning it into compassion, but the fact that this is a mere superficial antidote can be seen in the quantity of compassion that is necessary. The surplus of compassion testifies to the fear of a profound otherness, an otherness that cannot be interpreted as anything else than the face of an unacceptable loss.

The Linguistic Borders of Normality

The normality of one's own world is maintained not only through a surplus of compassion, but through the negativity of attack. Sighted people and blind people share a linguistic world, the English language, in which the borders of sighted totality are continually reinforced by linguistic difference. The metaphorical negativity defends against existential contrast by offering linguistic contrast. Organic theories of language emphasize that words gain their meaning not from those objects in the world to which they ostensibly refer, but from the distinction, the difference, between words. I recognize this because it is not that. So the English language reinforces the normality of sight by contrasting it with the negativity of blindness. Analyses of the vocabulary of blind and blindness in the daily newspapers reveals that nearly half of all cases are metaphors in which blindness is equated with stubbornness, indifference, insensitivity and ignorance. 'The Prime Minister shows a blind disregard for the welfare of this nation.' 'He struck out in blind fury.' 'They were blindly hostile to those who tried to help them.' Not only are such expressions to be found in almost every newspaper, every day, not only are they a part of the idiomatic vigour of everyday speech, but they are also normal within professional circles, so normal as to be virtually unnoticed. As noted earlier, medical researchers speak of carrying out a blind trial; examiners speak of blind marking. Such expressions depend upon the common view that blindness is a state of ignorance; they not only depend upon it, they reinforce it, and all who use such expressions collaborate with the negativity. Through thousands of repetitions, this rhetoric of abuse builds up the unconscious, taken-for-granted normality of the sighted world. The contrast between blindness and sight in our language continually reassures sighted people that to be sighted means to be sensible, knowledgeable, judicious, rational, while to be blind is to be the opposite of such qualities. Blind people also use this language, and thus unconsciously internalize the low self-esteem which the language reproduces.

Disability Awareness and Culture

It is regrettable that the language of faith and worship collaborates with this prejudice; indeed the Bible itself is a principal source of such negativity.[6] Even Jesus is reported to have used the word 'blind' as a term of abuse (Matt. 23.16–19, 24–26), and in the hymnbooks it is the sinful, the heathen, the idolaters and the unconverted who are blind (see Chapters 9 and 10 in this book). It is precisely because such language is metaphorical that it is so persuasive.

---

6 J. M. Hull, *In the Beginning There Was Darkness: A Blind Person's Conversations with the Bible*, London: SCM Press, 2001.

But is not the metaphor based upon accurate observation? Is it not true that blind people are ignorant and insensitive, clumsy and indiscriminating? Whether blind people are like this depends upon the situation, the point of view and the detail. A blind person would certainly be a rather indiscriminating motorist but would not be blind at all on the telephone. A blind person is ignorant of facial expression but by the same token cannot be deceived by appearances. Blind people do become rather indifferent to reported details that necessarily lie outside their experience. I listen with patient interest to my friend describing a stained glass window or a painting. My interest is just as much in the reactions and observations of my friend as it is in the object of description. Of course, blind people differ from each other as much as sighted people do. While it is true that blind people cannot do anything that sighted people cannot do, it may be the case that blindness enables tactile and acoustic experiences to be absorbed with greater concentration and intensity. At any rate, we certainly cannot compare the experiences of sighted and blind people point by point in this way, especially if we are coming from a philosophy of normality that assumes a deficiency model of disability. The Bible speaks of blindness as a curse from God (Acts 13.6–11) or as a metaphor of unbelief (John 9.39–41). It speaks of those who, being blind, lead other blind people into trouble (Matt. 15.14), but never refers to the skilful hands of the blind weaver or the blind potter. On the other hand, the Bible also takes blindness as a metaphor of faith, for 'we walk by faith not by sight' (2 Cor. 5.7) and faith itself is 'the evidence of things unseen' (Heb. 11.1). Not until the ambiguity of the religious and linguistic traditions is more vividly realized will the unconscious reinforcement of the exclusive world of normality be qualified.

The Learning Curve

The presuppositions, experiences and attitudes that I have described must represent significant educational barriers between sighted teachers and blind, or visually impaired, children. Indeed, in so far as my comments may be generalized across the whole field of handicap, we are dealing with a barrier between teachers who live average or normal lives, and students who do not. It is an educational barrier because there can be no genuine dialogue between a totalized world and that which is deemed to lie beyond it. The problem is not the normality as such, which nobody denies, but the tendencies toward absoluteness. Elements that are not comprehended by the totalized world must be thought of as out of place. Whether from an existential point of view in securing positive learning relationships between teachers and pupils, or whether from a more instrumental and vocational perspective, these obstacles must be overcome.

Mere human sympathy is insufficient. The sympathy that does not challenge the absolute character of the totalized world must turn into a condescending or patronizing attitude, into the desire to help or into a benevolence that simply fails to understand, or into pity. Even curriculum is involved, for how can a world create a curriculum for that other which it does not recognize as either being a world in itself or as being included within its own world?

Relating to Impaired and Disabled Children

We must carefully consider the character of each impairment, the autobiography of each child, and the kind of social and cultural context within which the child has developed. A world, in the sense we have been using it, is partly a creation of a physical or mental impairment which leads the child to experience life and the environment in a very different way, and partly a question of the extent to which the individual has been able to assemble the diverse experiences of living into a coherent body/world event. The temperament of the child, the degree to which simple philosophical, religious or spiritual nurture may have helped or hindered this process, and the way the child has responded to the attitudes of others towards its impairment will all have played a part. Each of these elements constitutes a continuum. For example, to lose one's hair, to go bald, is a loss and perhaps an embarrassment in the normal hairy-headed society, but it is probably not so extreme or distinct in the experiences it produces as to be called a world. Baldness is an attribute that may be possessed without causing one to transfer to a different world. To lose one's teeth or a finger may be somewhat similar, but to lose both one's arms or to be born without arms or without legs is so profoundly different that it might suggest the creation of a distinct world. Visual impairment takes many forms, and the experience of the totally blind may be radically different from those who are only partially sighted. There is a difference between using low-vision aids to maintain one's grasp upon the visual world and becoming a non-visual person.

Those who have reflected about the nature of blindness range from those who regard it as a mere characteristic and not as constituting a distinct human state, to those who emphasize its relative autonomy.

However, unless the possibility of living in concrete and integrated human worlds is recognized, the likelihood of there being a path consisting of many steps gradually leading into that world will also be disregarded. If many of the limitations and frustrations of teaching children spring from the difficulty that many adults have in entering into the world of childhood, it is not surprising that those who are in daily contact with children who not only inhabit the world of childhood but also the world of autism, deafness, blindness or other radically impaired conditions find them difficult to communicate with. The problem is not in the first instance pedagogical. It is ontological (belonging to what really is) and epistemological (having to do with the nature and grounds of knowledge). It involves having insight into a different human world, a world in which the nature of knowledge, what is taken to be knowledge, what is regarded as being important or unimportant knowledge, may be different from the one in which the teacher lives.

The Teacher as a Trans-World Professional

However, we should not despair. The many human worlds remain human. Most of us with experience, familiarity and imagination can enter adequately into the lives of another human being.

The teacher who can enter into several worlds will become a trans-world professional, and to that extent, a better teacher.

Acknowledgements of Previous Publication

'The Tactile Heart', *Expository Times* 102:10 (1991), pp. 311–12.

'The Material Spirituality of Blindness and Money', in Ruth Harvey (ed.), *Wrestling and Resting: Exploring Stories of Spirit from Britain and Ireland*, London: CTBI, 1999, pp. 69–72.

'Open Letter from a Blind Disciple to a Sighted Saviour: Text and Discussion', in Martin O'Kane (ed.), *Borders, Boundaries and the Bible*, Sheffield: Sheffield Academic Press, 2001, pp. 154–77.

'Blindness and the Face of God: Toward a Theology of Disability', in Hans-Georg Ziebertz *et al.* (eds), *The Human Image of God*, Leiden: Brill, 2000, pp. 215–29.

'A Spirituality of Disability: The Christian Heritage as Both Problem and Potential', *Studies in Christian Ethics* 16:2 (2003), pp. 21–36.

'The Broken Body in a Broken World: A Contribution to a Christian Doctrine of the Person from a Disabled Point of View', *Journal of Religion, Disability & Health* 7:4 (2003), pp. 5–23.

'"Sight to the Inly Blind"? Attitudes to Blindness in the Hymnbooks', *Theology* CV:827 (2002), pp. 333–41.

'"Lord, I was Deaf": Images of Disability in the Hymnbooks', in Stephen Burns, Nicola Slee and Michael Jagessar (eds), *The Edge of God, New Liturgical Texts and Contexts in Conversation*, Peterborough: Epworth, 2009, pp. 117–34.

'Teaching as a Trans-world Activity', *Support for Learning*, August 2004, pp. 103–6.

www.ingramcontent.com/pod-product-compliance
Lightning Source LLC
Chambersburg PA
CBHW051402290426
44108CB00015B/2115